Health and Wholeness for Clergy: Caring for Yourself and Your Congregation

Health and Wholeness for Clergy: Caring for Yourself and Your Congregation

by

Miguel A. Albert
D. Min.

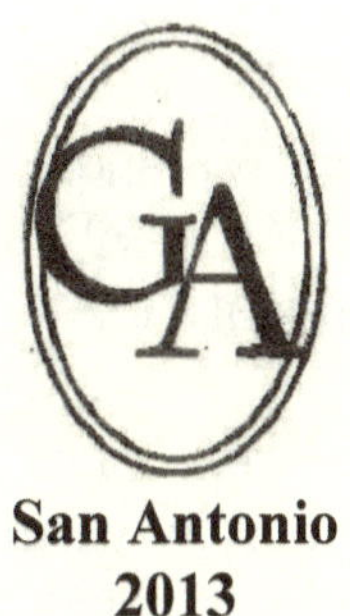

San Antonio
2013

A *Watercress Press* book
from Geron & Associates
www. watercresspress.com

ISBN-13: 978-0934955-94-2

NOTES ON SOURCES

Unless otherwise noted, Scripture taken from HOLY BIBLE INTERNATIONAL VERSION®. Copyright © 1973, 1978, 1984, by International Bible Society. Used by permission of Zondervon Publishing House. All rights Reserved

Saudek, Christopher D., M.D., Richard R. Rubin, Ph.D., and Cynthia S. Shump, R.N., *The Johns Hopkins Guide to Diabetes: For Today and Tomorrow.* pp. 29, 113, 116, 126, 139, 140. © 1997 The Johns Hopkins University Press. Reprinted with permission of The Johns Hopkins University Press.

Chasnoff, Ira J., Ellis, Jeffery W., and Fainman, Zachary. (1983). *Family Medical & Medical Guide.* P. 66. 1993. Lincolnwood, IL: By permission from © Publications International Ltd.

Extract from *Managing Your Mind: The Mental Fitness Gui*de by Gillian Butler and Tony Hope reprinted by permission of Peters Fraser &Dunlop (www.petersfraserdunlop.com) on behalf of Gillian Butler.

Acknowledgements

I would like to extend my gratitude to all those who gave me encouragement and support to write this book. Specifically, I would like to thank Bishop Joel N. Martinez, retired Bishop of the United Methodist Church, for giving me the opportunity to write this book, which started out as a simple project for clergy in the Rio Grande and Southwest Texas Conference. To Rev. Dr. Austin Frederick Jr., Ordained Elder of the Southwest Texas Conference of the United Methodist Church and Vice President of Pastoral Care Services, Methodist Healthcare System, San Antonio, Texas, for reviewing my manuscript and giving me valuable feedback and input, and also for his encouragement to publish this book.

I would also like to acknowledge Dr. Antonio Falcon, Director of the Family Health Center, Rio Grande City, Texas, member of US and Mexico Border Health Commission and nonvoting member of (CDC) Center for Disease Control, and Dr. Sergio Rodriguez, Medical Director of the Family Health Center, Rio Grande City, Texas, with whom I consulted on medical matters in Part Three of this book. Their input, feedback, and advice were very helpful to me.

Also, I would like to thank Mr. Jody Pedroza, NASM* Certified Professional Trainer and Senior Fitness Manager of Gold's Gym at Bandera Trail in San Antonio, Texas, who reviewed Part Three, the section on exercise and fitness, and gave me his expert advice and feedback.

A special thanks to Fabian G. Perez for providing me with the exercise photos on pages 87-96. I am deeply grateful for his contribution to this work.

Finally, yet importantly, I want to acknowledge my wife for her patience and the support and encouragement she gave me as I worked on my book project.

I am very grateful and indebted to all of you. God bless all of you.

---

*NASM: National Academy of Sports Medicine

CONTENTS

Health and Wholeness for Clergy:

Caring for Yourself and Your Congregation

Foreword

Health and Wholeness for Clergy: Caring for Yourself and Your Congregation, is a must-read for clergy and laity who are engaged in ministry with congregations or any other ministerial setting. It is the premise of this book that if pastors (clergy members) are to have healthy congregations they themselves must be healthy, lest they become "wounded healers" (if I may borrow a phrase from the ancient Greek legend of Asclepius, a physician who was himself a wounded healer). I write this book out of my own experience as a pastor and former district superintendent, working with lay and clergy members in the local church and district, and as a Chaplain-Clinician at the Methodist Specialty and Transplant Hospital in San Antonio, Texas, working with staff, patients, and their families. It also stems from my own needs for health and wholeness as I serve the people in the ministry to which I have been appointed.

This book is about health in three dimensions: mind, body, and spirit. I begin with an introduction in which I address the need for health and wholeness for clergy in order that they may care first and foremost for themselves, and then be able to care for the people in the congregation or ministerial setting where they have been appointed. To be healthy is one thing and to have wholeness is another. The difference between the two is found in the introduction where health and wholeness are defined. Health as we know is the absence of illness – whether in the physical, emotional, or spiritual aspect, while wholeness is the sum of these three. In other words, to have wholeness there needs to be harmony or a balance in health among the physical, mental/emotion, and spiritual. If the balance is lost, one cannot reach a state of wholeness.

In Part One: Spiritual Health, I write about the need for clergy to lead from the spiritual center, leading with their hearts rather than their heads. One important thing for ministers is to live a spiritually centered life, focused on the presence of God and leading the congregation to the place where God is calling them to be. It is highly important that pastors live a life of devotion to God through worship, prayer, reading of the Scripture, and participation in the sacraments, if they are to lead from the spiritual center of the congregation. Toward the end of Part One, I have included a helpful guide for weekly Scripture reading using the lectionary readings, which can also be helpful in preparing for Sunday worship and sermon.

Part Two: Mental Health, focuses on the mental emotional aspect of health. It deals with some of the baggage that some clergy carry around in their emotional backpacks, which can keep them from having an effective ministry. Among other matters, I address the topic of shame and guilt, indebtedness, stress, and the importance of time management. I have included some advice for clergy who are struggling emotionally and have realized that unless they get help they risk the opportunity of having an effective ministry.

Part Three is Physical Health, where I address the health issues such as obesity and its association with other health problems like diabetes, hypertension, and the risk of a stroke or heart attack. I also include a section on diet and exercise as a way to control diabetes and hypertension by losing weight. I dedicate a good portion of this final section to the importance of getting started with an exercise program that will contribute to weight loss and good health. There are some exercises which you can do at home or in a gym. Some photos have been included illustrating these exercises. They have worked for me and I know that if you get into a daily discipline of diet and exercise you too can enjoy a life of health and wholeness.

It is my hope that you read this book and recommend it to others so that you can enjoy the benefits of being healthy in body, mind, and spirit.

INTRODUCTION

HEALTH AND WHOLENESS DEFINED

When we speak of "health and wholeness", we often think of total and perfect physical health or the absence of any disease, infection, or illness in a person. These two words are so closely related that they almost seem synonymous. The Greeks have two words that relate to health: σώτήρία (sotería) and σώζώ (sózo). These words can be applied to the physical, spiritual, mental/emotional aspect of healing, depending on the context in which they are used. σώτήρία (Sotería) appears 57 times in the Greek New Testament, 50 in reference to salvation (spirit), three in reference to liberation (mind), and four in reference to physical health (body). σώζώ (Sózo) appears 109 times, 102 in reference to salvation (spirit), four in reference to physical health (body), and twice in reference to liberation (mind).[1]

We must be cognizant of the fact that no matter how many times these two words appear in the New Testament, they refer to a holistic healing: the healing of body, mind, and spirit. When there is a balance in spiritual, mental, and physical health, we can say that a person has health and wholeness. God intends for all human beings to have healthy bodies, minds, and spirits. God desires for every one of God's children to reach a state of health and wholeness in life.

The Merriam-Webster's Collegiate Dictionary gives the following definition of health:

> 1*a* **:** the condition of being sound in body, mind, or spirit; *especially***:** freedom from physical disease or pain *b* **:** the general condition of the body <in poor *health*> <enjoys good *health*> [1]

According to this definition, health relates to the physical or emotional state of the human body at any given moment. We are either in a poor physical state, or in good physical condition. We can be in a

---

[1] By permission, from *Merriam-Webster's Collegiate© Dictionary, 11th Edition* ©2013 by Merriam-Webster, Inc. (www.Merriam-Webster.com)

poor mental state, or mentally balanced. Similarly, we can be in poor spiritual condition, or we can be in a healthy spiritual state enjoying the fullness of life.

That same dictionary defines whole as follows;

> *1 a (1)*: free of wound or injury: UNHURT *(2)* : recovered from a wound or injury : RESTORED *(3)* : being healed . . . *b* : free of defect or impairment : INTACT *c* : physically sound and healthy : free of disease or deformity *d* : mentally or emotionally sound . . . 3 *a* : constituting the total sum or undiminished entirety : ENTIRE <owns the *whole* island> [2]

Parting from this definition, it is my understanding that to be whole one's entire being must be in good health. Thus we must have good physical health and be in sound mental and emotional state. I would add that since we, as human beings, were created by God who formed us "in his own image" (Genesis 1:27) and gave us a human body, and a mind to know "good and evil" (Genesis 3:22), to think and make our own decisions, and breathed in us spirit of life. We are therefore made up of body, mind, and spirit. These three are inseparable in every human being and need to be in harmony. That is to say; if we are to reach a state of wholeness, there needs to be a balance among these three elements. This means that we need to have healthy bodies, mind, and spirit if we are to reach a state of health and wholeness.

I am sure that you may have heard someone say at one time or another, "I have not had to see a doctor in many years because there is not a thing wrong with me. I am perfectly healthy." The truth is that a person can consider him or herself physically healthy, for the simple reason that the body is free of any injury, disease, infection or any other illness. However, if conditions between the body, mind, and spirit are not equally balanced, there can be no wholeness, as these three elements need to work in harmony and function as a system.

---

[2] By permission, from *Merriam-Webster's Collegiate© Dictionary, 11th Edition* ©2013 by Merriam-Webster, Inc. (www.Merriam-Webster.com)

In linear thinking, we think in terms of cause and effect where one thing can have influence on another thing and cause it to react accordingly

In systems thinking, according to Peter L. Steinke and other systems theory proponents, we look at elements in terms of the mutual influence in parts and how each element relates to the other, whereas, "Every cause has an effect; and every effect is a cause."[2] In other words, one thing can have influence over another while at the same time be reciprocally influenced by that very thing that caused the effect. In terms of health and wholeness, when something is wrong with our physical well-being it affects our mental and spiritual health. Similarly, when something is wrong with our mental/emotional well-being, both our spiritual and physical health can be affected, because each element influences and is mutually influenced by the other. And when our physical well-being is affected both our mental/emotional and spiritual health are affected as well, and so on. When there is a loss of balance in a system, it will cease to function properly. Like any other system, the body, mind, and spirit need to be in harmony in order to function properly. In the case of clergy members, a loss of balance in the system could affect the way they function within their family and church. This could easily affect their relationships with their family and church members to the detriment of their ministry, thus risking the possibility of having an effective ministry in the particular community where he or she has been called to serve.

Health and wholeness are therefore necessary for clergy members if they are to function properly and be effective in ministry. That is why it is important for pastors to care for themselves while caring for their congregations. That means taking care of our health in three dimensions: spirit, mind, and body.

PART ONE:

SPIRITUAL HEALTH

> *Everyone who competes in the games goes into strict training. They do it to get a crown that will not last; but we do it to get a crown that will last forever. Therefore, I do not run like a man running aimlessly; I do not fight like a man beating the air. No, I beat my body and make it my slave . . .*
> (1 Corinthians 9: 25-27)

Having defined health in the spiritual, mental/emotional, and physical dimensions, let us now consider how each element can affect our ministries and what we need to do to reach a state of health and wholeness for ourselves and our congregation. For Christians, especially clergy members, spiritual health should rank first on their list of priorities. In his book, *An Adventure in Healing and Wholeness*, James K. Wagner quotes David Hilton, M.D., in his address to 117th annual meeting of the American Public Health Association (October 24, 1989):

> . . . The most important dimension to health is the spiritual. Even in the midst of poverty, some people stay well, while among the world's affluent many are chronically ill. Why? Medical science is beginning to affirm that one's beliefs and feelings are the ultimate tools and powers for healing. Unresolved guilt, anger, resentment and meaninglessness are found to be the greatest suppressors of the body's powerful, health-controlling immune system, while loving relationships in community are among its strongest augmenters. Those in harmony with the Creator, the earth and their neighbors not only survive tragedy and suffering best but also grow stronger in the process. [3]

Perhaps you have heard the old cliché, "If you want things to go well, just get the spiritual things in order, and the rest will fall into place." There is no doubt in my mind that taking care of the spiritual order is the most important thing in life. More important than a good job, social status, material possessions or human prosperity, is the need for a relationship with God. Through that relationship we can have a spiritually enriched life. When we begin to live a life in the spirit, we learn to function in such a way that even in the midst of poverty we can stay well. While many people in this world have wealth, social status, and far more possessions than they need, they may lack spiritual and physical health. Nevertheless, those who seek first the kingdom of God and its righteousness can be counted among those who have been blessed with spiritual and physical wellness. We may not be among the world's most affluent people, and we may not even possess all the things that we would like to have, but we are "rich according to God's riches in glory."

One morning, while watching a talk show on the FOX News Station, I heard a physician say that Christians have a better chance of recovering from surgery or any serious illness than people who do not profess a Christian faith. We can say, therefore, that good health is not attributed to having large sums of money as much as it is to having a strong belief in God and a good Christian attitude toward life's situation. In Matthew 9:1-8, we read the story of a man taken to Jesus on a stretcher so that he could be healed. Jesus did not declare him healed right away. Instead, He dealt with the man's spiritual condition by declaring him forgiven of his sins. Jesus said to the man, "Take heart, son; your sins are forgiven." (Matthew (9:2) As you can see, Jesus wanted this man to put his spiritual life in order first. He pardoned the man's sins and then healed him physically, restoring him to wholeness.

In the Gospel according to Saint Mark, Chapter 5, we have the story of a woman who came to Jesus for healing. This woman had been suffering from a serious condition for more than twelve years. She had gone to various healers, but her condition had not improved. When she had exhausted all of her resources and realized that she could not be cured of her illness, she then turned to Jesus. She believed that if only she could get close to Jesus and touch the hem of his cloak, she would be saved. This woman appeared to have had her priorities in order. She wanted to be restored to wholeness by first being saved (spiritual healing) and then being cured (physical healing). When she touched the hem of Jesus' cloak, He turned around to see who had touched him. Though many people had touched him as he passed, he reacted to the touch of this woman; a special touch could not be overlooked. It was this woman's touch of faith that made Jesus unleash his power to heal.

But Jesus kept looking around to see who had done it. Then the woman, knowing what had happened to her, came and fell at his feet and, trembling with fear, told him the whole truth. He said to her. "Daughter, your faith has healed you. Go in peace and be freed from your suffering." (Mark 5:32-34)

Notice that this woman had spent her money on physicians and healers because she believed that if she went to the right one, they might find a cure for her condition. However, when she realized that they could do nothing for her condition, she turned her belief into faith in Jesus Christ, not just for physical healing, but primarily for the healing of her soul. She wanted to be restored to wholeness. (In the original Greek text the word *heal* in this context, means wholeness.) This woman had her priorities right. She thought about putting her spiritual life in order, and when she did, she received spiritual healing through the forgiveness of her sins; because of her faith physical healing took place. Like this woman, many people place their trust in the men and women of science and the medical means of healing. Nevertheless, medical science has its limitations, but Jesus' power to heal is without limits or boundaries. If we go to Jesus with faith he will release that healing power and bring forth healing and wholeness to our lives.

Leading From a Spiritual Center

If pastors are to be effective in ministry, they need to lead from the spiritual center of the congregation. By this I mean that pastors should live a spiritual life centered in Jesus Christ, knowing that their lives and the ministries to which they have been called all belong to God. We as ministers depend on God for all we do in God's name. We depend on God for salvation and direction for our lives. We also depend on the power of the Holy Spirit for the work of ministry; no one can do God's work without the power of the Holy Spirit. Leading from the spiritual center of the congregation means that all we do has to be for the glory and honor of God and not for self-aggrandizement or satisfaction of our personal interest. Leading from the spiritual center means doing what God directs us to do, rather than take the course we desire for our congregation and ourselves. Leading from the spiritual center means doing what pleases God, not the people. To lead from the spiritual center one must choose to live a life focused on Jesus Christ, "the author and finisher of our faith."

As pastors, we are open letters read by our congregations and people in our communities. Consequently, we have to live an exemplary life that can witness to Jesus Christ wherever we go, and not just when we gather in the congregation sharing in worship and fellowship with our brethren. What matters most to people is not so much what we say, but what we do. They expect our lives to shine with the light of Christ when we walk into a room.

Congregational leaders, church members, and people in the surrounding community often turn to pastors to seek spiritual advice. They see the pastor as a representative of Jesus Christ. They expect the pastor to be in close relationship with God, totally consecrated to the work of ministry, and expect them to bring a message from God that brings hope and gives new meaning and healing to their lives in the midst of their situations. A congregation's expectations and demands of the pastor are overwhelming. Some people actually see pastors as people who are perfect and blameless before God, flawless and infallible, incapable of being touched or affected by temptation, sin, and evil. However, we are human as humans can be, and as such we are vulnerable and capable of being affected spiritually, physically, and emotionally. We are prone to all kinds of suffering, pain, illness, and disease, and even death can come to any one of us when we least expect it.

In a congregation I once served, a parishioner heard from our lay leader that I would not be at the evening service because I had come down with a bad case of bronchitis. After a few days of dealing with pain and discomfort caused by this bronchial infection, I was able to get back on my feet. On the following Sunday, that same parishioner said to me, "Pastor, I am so glad that you are back today and feeling better. However, I do have to tell you that I was surprised to hear that you were sick. I never expected that something like that could happen to you, a man of God." To that I responded, "Why should it surprise you? I am only human."

Staying in the Spiritual Center

Staying in that spiritual center takes discipline and hard work. It takes determination and dedication to the spiritual discipline of prayer, Scripture reading, devotion, and a strong commitment to God and our call to ministry. It involves taking care of ourselves spiritually so that we can care for and nurture the people in our congregations as we journey together. I use the term "journey" because it best describes our walk with God and God's people as we travel together in faith, experiencing spiritual renewal and a deeper understanding of Jesus Christ and his plan and purpose for each of us. In this journey, it is Jesus leading the way as we move forward in life in our journey of faith. Paul seems to be talking about the Christian journey as we move on forward in life and continue our journey to our final destination, the kingdom of God, which is our ultimate goal. Paul says that the way he can attain this is by ". . . Forgetting what is behind and straining toward what is ahead, I press on toward the goal to win the prize for which God has called me heavenward in Christ Jesus" (Philippians 3:13-14). As we walk together in this journey of faith, we pray to God for strength hoping to be able to reach the finish line.

As spiritual leaders, pastors are in the public eye of the people in our community. They look to us for direction and advice because they trust that God is with us always, 24/7. They seem to think that we have a direct line to God. For this reason, pastors need to stay in the spiritual center focusing and leading others to focus on the presence of God. Nevertheless, focusing constantly on God is not easy. It takes hard work and discipline. Michael Slaughter, author of *Momentum for Life*, says:

> In the same way, God is always speaking, but we are not always present to the relationship. Does it ever seem to you like God is hiding? The real problem is that we are the ones who are not aware of God's presence. Devotion is a time of being present to God's presence. This becomes both hard work and intentional discipline. [4]

Pastors often find themselves trying to keep up with their busy schedules, working 60 to 70 hours a week; which barely gives them time to focus intentionally on the presence of God. A few of my colleagues with whom I have talked about this subject have confessed that they often leave for work without morning devotions because they are on such a tight schedule. One quick prayer and they are off to work, trying to get to their office early to catch up on work left behind from the previous day. Some may log onto their computers, check e-mail, and respond before doing a hospital visit here and a home visit there. Life comes at them so fast that they have to take advantage of any opportunity that comes along to read the Scripture in preparation for Sunday morning worship. Some pastors get so busy with administrative work, programs, counseling, and visitation that they very seldom take time for their families.

Pastors can become, in a sense, "wounded healers," caring for others without taking time to care for their selves. Many pastors try to solve other people's problems while putting theirs to one side. Some go as far as trying to mend somebody else's marriage while their own might be falling apart. When wounded healers see someone going through pain and suffering, they put aside their own needs to tend to the needs of others. Wounded healers want to take care of their congregations, while neglecting their own health and well-being and that of their family. While attempting to help others work out their problems, they often forget that they too have problems that they need to take care of and a family that needs their love, support, and attention.

When ministers become so bogged down in their ministry and fail to take time from their busy schedule to care for their own needs and the needs of their loved ones, they risk burnout and loss of focus on the presence and purpose of God in their lives. When this happens, it is time to take a break and go into a quiet place where they can be alone in silence in the presence of God. When we find ourselves completely alone with God in discernment and prayer, and opened to what the Spirit has to say to us, we may hear the voice of God speaking to our mind and soul as God renews our spirit.

As ministers, we need to remain at the spiritual center by making God our first priority and always maintaining our focus on the power and presence of God, who guides, directs, sustains, and strengthen us in our ministry. This can only be achieved when we dedicate ourselves to the practice of daily spiritual discipline.

Spiritual Disciplines

Before athletes compete, they work hard to get into shape, in order to be fit for their athletic event. They live a disciplined life, abstaining from all things that might affect their health and performance. They submit to a healthy diet and exercise program that will get their bodies in shape and in optimum condition for the competition. In his first letter to the Corinthians Paul uses the analogy of the athlete to demonstrate the importance of a disciplined lifestyle:

> Do you not know that in a race all the runners run, but only one gets the prize. Run in such a way as to get the prize. Everyone who competes in the games goes into strict training. They do it to get a crown that will not last; but we do it to get a crown that will last forever. Therefore I do not run like a man running aimlessly; I do not fight like a man beating the air. No, I beat my body and make it my slave . . . (1 Corinthians 9: 24-27)

Paul's idea of living a disciplined lifestyle implies denying the body of the pleasures that his flesh desires. He submits to such standards obediently. The athlete does that to strengthen his body so that he can win the competition. The Christian lives a disciplined life to strengthen his/her spirit so he or she can win the battle against sin and evil. The athlete needs proper diet and exercise to develop firm muscles. He needs to get the proper amount of sleep so that he can be mentally alert. Similarly, Christians need to submit to a spiritual discipline if they are to develop strong faith, firm convictions, sound mental alertness, and constant awareness of the presence of God. The Christian minister's daily discipline should include setting time aside for devotion, prayer, fasting, Scripture reading, and participation in the sacraments.

Devotion to God

"Devotion," Michael Slaughter says, "is what you ultimately care about, what you value." [5] Devotion is the one thing you value in life; dedicate your time to it with enthusiasm.

In the movie *Million Dollar Baby*, Maggie Fitzgerald (Hillary Swank) dreamed of becoming a professional boxer. Every day after work, she would go to a gym to practice on the speed bag. Day after day she would work out until the gym was about to close. She had hoped that Frank (Clint Eastwood) would take some time to train her, but he had no interest in that because he was a man who lived by many rules, and as a rule he did not train girls. Nonetheless, Maggie continued to practice every day, throwing punches at the bag. She continued to insist that Frank take some time to train her. One day after much insistence, Frank finally agreed to be her trainer, but under certain conditions. With much enthusiasm, she continued to practice hard. She would go to the gym every day and stay until closing time. Then, one day after much practice, Frank felt that she was fit and ready to go professional. Therefore, he set up a few contracts for her, and after she had won several bouts, Frank felt that she was now ready for a shot at the title that would make her a "Million Dollar Baby." Maggie's passion for the sport and her deep desire to become a professional boxer got her into the daily workout discipline, which paid off in full.

As Christians, we need to understand the importance of living a Christ-centered life. We need to live fully focused on the presence of God. However, that is not always an easy task. It takes dedication, enthusiasm, and a strong commitment to God and our call to ministry. This takes much sacrifice and dedication to God through fasting, prayer, and service. To do this, we must live a purpose-driven life and a willingness to go the distance in order to grow in faith and strengthen our spirit; and in so doing, we can achieve spiritual health and wholeness as we grow from grace to grace.

Devotion and Prayer

Daily devotion is what we do in the presence of God. It is our time together with the Lord, as we praise and honor his name and render ourselves to God in worship and prayer. Devotion and prayer are inseparable. A life of devotion and prayer renews our spirit; gives us meaning, purpose, direction for life, and strengthens us to perform our daily tasks and meet our daily challenges. Devotion should be the first thing we do each day, which means that we need to rise early in the morning to find a quiet place where we can spend some quality time alone with God.

Jesus made devotion his first priority every morning. In Mark 1:35 we see Jesus getting up early to make his way to a quiet place to begin his daily devotion and prayer. Even before the sun would rise on the horizon, Jesus rose from his bed and made his way out of the house and into a quiet place where he spent some time alone in devotion and prayer before starting his day. In so doing, He found strength and empowerment for the challenges that he would encounter throughout the day. There is no mention in the gospels as to how long Jesus remained in that lonely place or how he prayed, but we can surmise that he was deeply engaged in fervent prayer in the presence of God.

We learn from Mark 1:35 the importance of starting our day alone, in a place of solitude, in devotion and prayer with God, asking God to give us strength and courage, as we prepare to meet our daily challenges. Jesus demonstrated to us the crucial importance of putting first things first. The word solitude is derived from the Latin word *solus*. But we do not need to run off to some remote, isolated place in order to find solitude. There, in our own home, we can find a quiet place where we can spend some quiet time alone in silence and in the presence of God. In the midst of silence, we can hear the sweet gentle voice of God as God tries to speak to us.

I sometimes encounter difficulty in praying when I have too many things on my mind. However, when I get up early in the morning the first thing I do is try to empty my mind of all worries and concerns. I do that by thinking about my present priority and realizing that unless I begin my day with prayer, I will not be able to accomplish all that I set out to do. I begin by putting on a compact disk with praise music and closing my eyes to meditate on the words of the song. This prepares me to focus on prayer and on the presence of Jesus Christ. While the music is playing, I begin to praise God until I get into a spirit of prayer. Not just any simple prayer where there is lip movement with words pouring out one after the other without meaning, but with words that come from the heart with profound meaning, that elevate the mind and spirit to the throne of grace, before the presence of God.

We begin our prayer and devotion by first emptying ourselves of all worries and concerns and seeking the presence of God with all our mind, heart, and strength. We need to pour our souls out to God in prayer and adoration. As we pray in this manner, the Holy Spirit takes over; and before you know it, we find ourselves submerged in fervent prayer in the Spirit, who will bring to our mind things to pray about and people for whom we need to pray. As we continue praying with our mind and spirit, we will begin to feel the presence of God in our lives and be able to tap into some of his strength, in such a way that will enable us to meet our challenges throughout the day.

Let us remember that without Christ, we can do nothing, and without the help of the Holy Spirit, we cannot do the work of God or be effective in ministry. We need to live a life of prayer and devotion with God; furthermore, we need to search the Scripture if we are to witness to God and show people the way of salvation.

Worship and Scripture Reading

Worship and Scripture reading can be done in community or individually. They instruct and edify the Christian minister and layperson. Worship and Scripture reading are means of grace by which we grow spiritually in our relations with God and with the Christian community. Worship involves rendering devotion and giving respect and adoration to God in the context of a religious service, where a Christian community is present. However, worship is not limited to rites in the presence of a large community, for there are two kinds of worship: *congregational* or *collective* and *individual* or *personal* worship.

Congregational or Collective Worship

In congregational or collective worship, a Christian community is present. A designated person leads the worship service with the use of a structured format that includes some standard elements such as, opening prayer, reading of a Psalm, responsive reading, congregational hymns, Scripture reading, offering, preaching, sacraments, closing prayer, benediction, and other things included by the pastor and worship committee. In the United Methodist Church this worship is all-inclusive. Any member of the congregation is able to participate. All who are present, whether members of the local church or visitors from other congregations, are welcome to receive the Eucharist. I conceive Sunday worship as a celebration of the mighty works of God in our lives. It is our way of thanking God and recognizing publicly what God has done in, for, and through us. What makes worship a religious or Christian service is that it is directed only to God, who is worthy of all honor, glory, and praise.

Individual or Personal Worship

Individual or personal worship, like collective worship, is directed to God. It is done in a more informal setting and without a formal structure, and can be done in the privacy of our home or office. Personal worship can include prayer, singing a hymn, Scripture reading from the Old and New Testament, Epistles, and Psalms. Readings can be done according to a theme you choose for the day. I often pick a theme from a devotional book such as *The Upper Room*, *Bread of Life,* or *Daily Disciplines*, from Discipleship resources, or I might read the lectionary text for the following Sunday and use it as part of my devotional reading.

There are different approaches to reading the Scripture. One of the ways is known as Contemplative Scripture reading which plays a very special role in our devotions. Through contemplative reading of Scripture, God can speak to us at any given moment and under any situation or circumstance that we may be facing. Reading Scripture can give us direction for the day and even lead us to a spiritual renewal of life. As a matter of fact, St. Augustine had his conversion experience when he responded to a child urging him to read the Scripture. The child was quoted as saying to him, "Take, and read. Take, and read." Augustine confessed that, "When he took the Bible and started reading the page on which he opened it; he felt that the words he read were directly spoken to him."

There have been times when I have found myself in situations where I have desperately sought advice and had no one to turn to. While engaging in a quiet time of devotion and silent prayer, I turned to the Scripture to do some contemplative reading and felt that through a particular passage God had spoken to me. When we dedicate some time to be in the presence of God in worship and prayer, and as we silently read Scripture and meditate on God's word, we become attentive to the "still small voice" as He speaks to our soul. When we engage in contemplative reading, God can speak to us in the midst of our needs and our situation in life.

Oftentimes, we want to hear the voice of God but do not take time to listen. There are other instances when our prayers become a monologue, a one-way conversation so that we keep ourselves from listening to God's voice wanting to speak to us. When we pray we need to take time out for a moment of silence and wait to hear what the Lord has to say to us. In the midst of our silence and patient waiting, we may be able to hear the still small voice of God speaking to us in ways never imagined.

Another way to read Scripture during our time of devotion is in a Bible study. This reading is different from contemplative reading. In contemplative reading the Bible talks to us, leading us to reflection and meditation. In a Bible study, Scripture informs us. It then allows us to take an exegetical approach to the text, asking it questions in order to extract its full meaning. As we analyze the text, we become informed about the history of God and God's people, and of how God continues to move in the world today to bring his redemptive act to fulfillment. In a Bible study, we do not just read Scripture as we would any other book. Instead, we study Scripture in search of God's promises, which give us hope of eternal life. Jesus said, "You diligently study the Scriptures because you think that by them you possess eternal life. These are the Scriptures that testify about me." (John 5:39) We study the Scripture because it points the way to God's kingdom and because it witnesses to our Lord Jesus Christ, the author of our salvation. We also search the

Scripture because it helps us to understand God and God's divine purpose with humankind.

As we read the Scripture, we not only increase our knowledge and understanding of God, but we grow from grace to grace as we abide by His word, do His will, and seek to live a life that is pleasing to God. God wants us to live the fullness of life: a life that is measured not by its longevity, but by how purposeful, intentional, and meaningfully we have lived our lives in the presence of God. The Bible therefore informs, inspires, and gives hope, meaning, and purpose to our lives as we make it part of our daily devotion.

We must vary in our personal morning devotional from time to time so as not to make it a routine but a discipline. A routine is something that you do automatically, not necessarily with a purpose or for creating meaning. You do it for the sake of not breaking the daily pattern. A routine cannot be interrupted or altered: if there is any change in what you are doing, the rhythm is broken. In a routine, there is no intentional purpose other than to repeat what you do day after day, causing you to fall into a vicious cycle of doing the same thing over and over, to the point where boredom sets in. On the other hand, a discipline has a meaningful purpose and is done with intentionality. A discipline can be interrupted. Once interrupted, you can pick up where you left off and continue from there. In a discipline, meaning can be created.

Design for Daily Devotional

To have a meaningful devotional you must design your personal worship around the time you are willing to invest. The time spent on this devotional is the best investment you will make during your day. Devotional time will get you off to a great start and carry you through the day. As you gradually work your way into this daily discipline, I suggest you open your devotional with a prayer thanking God for God's presence and for the many blessings that God has poured upon you, as you live from day to day. Ask God to prepare your mind, your heart, and your spirit as you start your devotional.

Proceed by reading a Psalm or a portion of a Psalm. Try repeating the verse that captures your attention and best speaks to your life. Read the verse a few times – once aloud, once in a low whisper, and once silently. Try memorizing the verse in such a way that you can repeat it throughout the day. Meditate for a few minutes on the verse and then remain quiet for a few minutes, trying to hear the voice of God speaking to you. Write down the first thought that comes to your mind. Did you feel that God spoke to you?

Now go before God in prayer. Begin with words of praise rather than just jumping immediately into your prayer request. Always begin by acknowledging God's presence, and exalting God for God's greatness and mighty works in your life. This will help to transition you into a spirit of prayer and discernment of God's presence. For prayer to be meaningful it must be intentional and purposeful. This can only happen when you become aware that as you pray God is present and listening. After all, did you ever try to have a conversation with a person who was not listening or a person who was not present? That conversation had no meaning or purpose whatsoever.

To speak to God, you need to perceive God as being present even though you cannot see God – for God is spirit. You can become consciously aware of God's presence and confident that God not only listens to prayer but that God will speak to you as well. Prayer can be a monologue or a dialogue. It can take the form of a monologue when we talk to God in prayer without awareness of God's presence and not taking time to listen and wait for a response. Prayer becomes a dialogue when we pray to God in faith, knowing that God is present listening to each word and ready to respond. Have you ever taken time after prayer to wait quietly and patiently to hear a word from God in answer to your prayer? Next time you pray open your heart, mind, and ears, and listen to the still small voice of God as God speaks to you. You might not be able to hear God's voice in an audible way, but if you are receptive to God's voice, God can speak to you in ways that you never imagined.

Once you have finished with your prayer of praise and thanksgiving and your prayer request, end your devotion by thanking God for honoring you with God's presence. Trust that God will answer your prayer according to God's will. If you believe this, get up and go in peace. Be confident that God will guide and lead you for the remainder of the day, and that the time that you have set aside for devotion and prayer has not been wasted, but has become an investment of time for which you will be compensated throughout the day. I once heard it mentioned in a Bible study group at church that the German reformer Martin Luther was a busy man but always made prayer the first priority on his list. When he got up early in the morning to start his day he would say, "I have so much to do today that I guess I will spend the next four hours in prayer."

Now that you have started and are feeling comfortable with a half hour of worship and prayer every morning, go one step further. Adjust your devotional time to one full hour. That will be a big challenge because we often get so comfortable doing something routinely that we very easily fall into our own comfort zones. Most ministers are constantly challenging their congregations to get out of their comfort zones. Comfort zones can lead us into a routine where there is no meaning and purpose, and with no room for growth. A routine can often make us do things mechanically just for the sake of doing whatever it is that we are doing. For this reason, pastors need to push the envelope, especially when it comes to our personal spiritual growth. It is like preparing for a sports competition. The athlete gradually needs to start an exercise program that will help develop strong muscles. He needs to practice techniques to increase his skills and enable him to qualify for the sports competition. After he has mastered the basic skills and developed strong muscles, he challenges himself to go the second mile by increasing his exercise to another level. Once he has accomplished this he will then be able to compete with confidence.

Increasing Daily Devotional Time

Your challenge now is to increase your daily devotional time by two. Instead of a half hour, you can now try increasing to one full hour of meaningful and intentional devotion to God. This will give you more time for prayer, Scripture reading, Bible study, sacraments, and other "means of grace," as described by John Wesley. Mr. Wesley referred to these as "means of grace" because as we participate in these practices, the grace of God is conveyed and made available to us.

I suggest that you make an effort to arise at the early hours of the morning, perhaps 6 a.m., when all is quiet, and make prayer and worship your first priority of the day. You can start by doing a half hour, then gradually work your way up to an hour, and perhaps even an hour and a half or so a day. The process may not be as easy as you may think. It may take some time to get into this discipline. As a matter of fact, there might be times when you find yourself struggling with boredom as you are saying the same thing over and over, waiting for time to go by fast, as you encounter resistance by spiritual forces that want to keep you from engaging in fervent prayer. Having too many things in your mind at this time can become a big distraction that could keep you from focusing on prayer. Nonetheless, you can overcome those obstacles simply by emptying your mind of all preoccupations and becoming totally focused, intentional, and purposeful in your devotion to God.

You need to realize that your time with God requires something more than just dropping to your knees and uttering the same words over and over again. The desire to become intentional in prayer can drive you to reflect on ways to approach God in prayer that is purpose driven and meaningful, not something done routinely. You need to realize that if you are going to be purposeful and intentional in your time with God, you need to be willing to invest rather than spend time before the Lord. When you spend time it is time that is gone forever, and you get nothing in return. On the other hand, when you invest quality time in the Lord that time will be compensated one way or another, and you will bear much fruits from your labor.

Parting from that premise, you can design a worship plan that can make your devotional time a more meaningful and interesting experience every time. It is important to remember that worship designs are not written on stone. You do have some recommended elements to use in worship, but the way you praise God can vary according to the situation and the context of the worshiping community.

I recommend that each morning when you get out of bed you find a place of solace where you can encounter the presence of God. If you have children who get up early to go to school, the time before they arise might work best for you. The earlier you start, the more time you will have available to do other things during the day. When you make prayer and praise your first priority, you will be better prepared for the challenges that you will encounter throughout the day. To invest quality time with God and make that moment meaningful, put all your heart, mind, and spirit into that moment. Your time alone with God should be one of the most special and meaningful events of the day. Therefore, you should not leave for work without having your time alone with God in devotional, prayer, moments of deep reflection on the word of God, and patiently waiting to hear the voice of God speaking to your heart and soul.

We live in a fast-moving world and life comes at you fast. On top of that, we have many responsibilities and demands placed on us by our families, church, and community. We barely have time for anything else. We live our lives worrying about time and commitments. We live by the clock and become a slave to time. We have so many things that keep our mind occupied and so many thoughts and worries which cause distractions in our lives. These distractions can occupy a space in our mind, keeping us from becoming consciously aware of God's presence. For this very reason, we need to empty our mind of any preoccupation, worries, or other thoughts that might keep us from concentrating whole-heartedly on the Lord. You will have plenty of time during the day to do all the things you need to do. You may even discover, as you invest time alone with God in worship and prayer, that your day will go by much more smoothly and you will be able to accomplish all that you set out to do.

As you prepare for your morning devotional, I recommend that you turn off the computer and leave it off until you have finished. There is always the temptation to check e-mail. Perhaps one message will be marked urgent. You will probably want to answer that one – and probably another. Before you know it, time has slipped through your fingers and that time you have wasted is gone forever.

Before you start your morning devotional, you may want to try this: insert a Christian music compact disk into your CD player and play it at a medium-low volume. This will often help you get started by clearing your mind and getting you into a spirit of praise and prayer. Close your eyes and concentrate on the words of the song. Listen for at least five to ten minutes – until you feel your mind is free and ready to focus totally on the presence of God. If you feel the spirit of God moving you to praise God, do so. As you continue to praise God, the Holy Spirit will guide you in your moment of devotion and prayer. At this time, you can proceed with a prayer of invocation, asking God to make you aware of God's presence that was there even before you started. After some time in prayer, follow up with a reading from *The Upper Room* or some other daily devotional resource. Many devotional resources contain inspirational readings that can lead you to a moment of deep reflection. Once you have reflected, take time to listen to what God has to say. You will be surprised to see the many different ways in which God can speak to your life. Offer a prayer of thanksgiving thanking God for all the things that he has done and continues to do in, for, and through you. End this prayer with words of "praise and an amen."

Make Scripture reading part of your devotional. This is very important because it enables God to speak to your needs and address your spiritual concerns. Using the lectionary as part of your devotion helps you in preparation for the Sunday worship service. As you follow the lectionary readings for Year A, B, and C, you will have read every major theme in the Bible in three years. There are four Scripture readings per Sunday beginning with a Psalm, Old Testament reading, a reading from an epistle, and a reading from the Gospel. Read and reflect on a different portion of the lectionary lesson each day.

Here is how your daily devotional Scripture reading should look for the week:

Monday – Read the Psalm in the lectionary for the following Sunday, but do not use commentaries at this time. Read it once silently, then a second time aloud. Read it a third time, looking for key words. Finally, look for a verse that catches your attention and ask the text some questions such as: What is the *sitz im leben* (the situation in the life of the church)? How is this situation similar to our situation today? How does this text address the issues in our church and community today? What is God calling us to do in the midst of the situation? How will I respond to this call? After answering these questions write a final thought and end with a prayer.

Tuesday – Read the Old Testament lectionary reading using the same technique as with the Psalm. Again, write your final thoughts and end with a prayer.

Wednesday – Read the Epistle and follow through with the same process as the Psalm and Old Testament reading.

Thursday – Repeat the exercise with the Gospel reading.

Friday – You can now read the commentaries and other exegetical and hermeneutical resources on each of the readings.

Saturday – Select the Scripture reading, illustrations and/or analogy that you will use for the sermon. Invest the rest of your time in preparation for your sermon for Sunday. Most of all, take time for prayer.

Your daily devotions during the week should serve not only for your personal spiritual edification, but it should also serve as a tool and a process for helping you minister effectively to the people in your congregation, and bring spiritual edification to their lives through the Word of God. As you continue to do this on a daily basis, you will be able to work yourself into a daily discipline, which will become second nature to you. You will also experience a healthy spiritual life, which will contribute to a balance between spiritual, mental, and physical health that will lead you to a life of health and wholeness.

PART TWO:

MENTAL HEALTH

I seek you with all my heart; do not let me stray from your commands. I have hidden your word in my heart that I might not sin against you. (Psalm 119:11)

A little over three decades ago, there was a slogan that read: "A mind is a terrible thing to waste." It was part of a public service campaign by the Ad Council for the United Negro College Fund (UNCF), encouraging Americans to give financial support. The intent was threefold: (1) to encourage African Americans across the United States to pursue an education beyond high school, (2) to encourage Americans to support the campaign, and (3) to make people aware of the need to help young African Americans further their education, so that they could make a measurable difference in their society. In an article posted in the internet titled UNCF (1972 – Present) we learn that since 1972, when this slogan was launched, the campaign has helped to raise more than $2.2 billion and has helped to graduate more than 350,000 minority students from 43 UNCF member colleges and universities. [6]

Thanks to this slogan that encouraged support to African Americans and other minorities, there are many opportunities for African Americans and other minorities in high-level, high-paying positions in this country.

The Human Mind

There are people today who still refer to the mind and the brain as one and the same. Mind and brain are very intimately related. Both exercise a function within our mental processes. However, they are not the same. The mind as defined in the *Encarta World English Dictionary* is:

> 1. SEAT OF THOUGHT AND MEMORY the center of consciousness that generates thoughts, feelings, ideas and perceptions and stores knowledge and memories. 2. THINKING CAPACITY capacity to think, understand, and reason (often used in combination) 3. CONCENTRATION concentration, or the ability to concentrate . . . [7]

The brain, on the other hand, is defined in that same dictionary as:

> 1. ANAT ORGAN OF THOUGHT AND FEELING the controlling center of the nervous system in vertebrates, connected to the spinal cord and enclosed in the cranium. It consists of a mass of nerve tissue and nerve-supporting and nourishing tissue (neuroglia), is the center of thought and emotions, and regulates bodily activities . . . [8]

By definition, the mind and brain exercise the same function as the center of thoughts, feelings, ideas and perceptions, and the storing of knowledge and memories. However, the brain is an organ, something that is observable, measureable, and quantifiable. It acts in a mechanical fashion coordinating movement of the different organs and body parts, transmitting and receiving information through electrical pulses, and then storing that data. We know that the brain is in the cranium and sends messages to the rest of the body through the nerves in the spinal cord.

The mind, on the other hand, is abstract. We can neither see nor feel it. Research continues on the mind. Some believe it is in the brain while others believe it resides in our conscience. Among Jews of the Old Testament world and during Jesus' time, the heart was considered the center of all thoughts and emotions. People believed the heart was the seat of the mind and conscience, the place where all perceived events and experiences were processed, registered, and permanently stored. They believed all human intelligence resided in the heart.

That is why the Psalmist wrote; "I have hidden your word in my heart that I might not sin against you." (Psalm 119:11) The author of Proverbs writes, "In his heart a man plans his course . . ." (Proverbs 16:9). In the book of Hebrews we read, "For the word of God is living and active. Sharper than any double-edge sword, it penetrates even to dividing the soul and spirit, joints and marrow; it judges the thoughts and attitudes of the hear.t" (Hebrews 4:12) Many Scriptures in the Old and New Testaments refer to the heart as the seat of the mind. The question is, can we actually pinpoint or assign a location to something that is abstract?

The United Negro College Fund advertising slogan from the 1970s implied that a mind was something that you could lose. The phrase "Use it or lose it" was also used in reference to the mind, but how can anyone lose something so abstract as the human mind, which is part of the human conscience and mental thought process. Robert Jarvik writes in the foreword of Marilyn vos Savant's book *Brain Building: Exercising Yourself Smarter*:

> Your mind is the heart of the spirit of your life. It is the one thing that can never be taken from you and the one thing that you can never give away. It is always yours, under your control, build it, and you build the workings of your future. Let it stagnate, and you live in the past. [9]

Our creator has gifted us with intellectual capacity and the ability to think, rationalize, and make our own decisions. However, when we come into this world our minds are like a tabula rasa, a clean slate with nothing written on it. Our minds begin to develop as we feel, see, and experience the world that surrounds us, through our sensory receptors. Experiences are then written on that clean slate as bits and blocks of information that help us to interpret, analyze, and understand the world in which we live. With every new piece of information written on the slate, we begin to expand our intellectual capacity and have a broader understanding of our world. What is written in our mind can never be lost. It stays with us forever. Our mind is ours from birth to death. We can neither lose our mind by giving it away, nor lose it by having someone take it from us. The slogan, "A mind is a terrible thing to waste," was used to encourage African Americans to take advantage of the educational opportunities that were being offered by the UNCF. Not taking advantage would imply that one's opportunity to expand one's knowledge would be a waste.

Mental Health

Mental health refers to the condition of a person's mind at any given moment. We can be either in a sound and healthy state of mind or in an unhealthy mental condition. Since the mind is something abstract and not measurable or perceivable with the human eye, we can only evaluate the state of a person's mental condition through the behavior or emotional patterns the person displays.

Mind and Emotions

The mind can generate different emotional states at different times depending on the situation that a person may be going through. These can be observed in the different moods that a person displays. They may be feeling jovial today and miserable tomorrow. On the other hand, there are also people who are always feeling miserable and talking negatively. Nothing ever seems right to them. They are constantly carrying a load of emotional baggage everywhere they go. Emotional baggage can manifest in a variety of ways, and cause the symptom bearer (the person displaying the behavior) to experience different attitudes or feelings such as guilt and shame, low self-esteem, feelings of inadequacy, unresolved personal or family issues, or even irrational fear. If these attitudes are left unattended because the person is in a state of denial or any other reason, the situation could get worse and lead to stress, anxiety, depression, or maybe even psychosis. Psychosis is the highest level of depression a person can reach. Psychosis often requires hospitalization. Any one of us could fall into these problems if we do not learn to cope with stress, tension or emotional instability.

Clergy members are not exempt from emotional baggage or levels of stress. However, they often have to differentiate by putting aside their emotions while preaching, counseling, or ministering to others. In so doing, they often become wounded healers. They hide their emotions from the members of the church and community for fear that others might see their personal struggles or emotions as a weakness. There may also be some pastors who seem to have a "Messiah complex." They feel that they have to fix the world's problems even while their own lives may be falling apart. This emotional baggage can often be a distraction for pastors in their ministries, which can lead them to frustration. For this reason, it is important to recognize the many ways emotional problems can surface, their causes, and their effects on the pastor and his or her ministry.

Shame and Guilt

The *Encarta World English Dictionary* defines shame as:

> 1. NEGATIVE EMOTION a negative emotion that combines feelings of dishonor, unworthiness, and embarrassment. 2. CAPACITY TO FEEL UNWORTHY the capacity or tendency to feel shame. . . *He has no shame* 3. STATE OF DISGRACE a state of disgrace or dishonor . . . . *Bring shame on the family*. . . [10]

The same dictionary defines guilt as:

> 1. AWARENESS OF WRONGDOING an awareness of having done wrong or committed a crime, accompanied by feelings of shame and regret or feelings of guilt 2. FACT OF WRONGDOING the fact of having committed a crime or done wrong . . . . *an admission of guilt* . . .[11]

Though shame and guilt, by definition, have different meanings, they are intimately related. One is the cause. The other is the effect. Guilt is produced by feelings people get when they become aware that they did something contrary to their beliefs and values. For example, a person taught that lying is wrong might feel guilty after telling a lie or giving misleading information. The person's conscience begins to bother him or her, to the point where feelings of unworthiness, dishonor, and embarrassment can be generated.

The difference between shame and guilt, according to John Bradshaw, author of *Healing the Shame That Binds You*, is that "while guilt is a painful feeling of regret and responsibility for one's actions, shame is a painful feeling about oneself as a person." [12] I agree with Bradshaw that shame can be a destructive force. It can affect us emotionally if we do not overcome it. Bradshaw confessed:

> Shame was the unconscious demon I had never acknowledged. In becoming aware of the dynamics of shame, I came to see that shame is one of the major destructive forces in all-human life. In naming shame, I began to have power over it. [13]

Though Bradshaw considers shame to be "one of the major destructive forces in all-human life," in my opinion it is not all that bad. Shame is part of the human emotional system and everyone lives with a certain degree of shame. Bradshaw further suggests that shame is necessary if we are to be truly human:

> In fact, it is necessary to have the feeling of shame if one is to be truly human. Shame is the emotion that gives us permission to be human. Shame tells us our limits . . . Our shame tells us that we are not God. [14]

Shame, therefore, is like an alarm. It makes us aware that we are not perfect human beings. "Shame," says Lewis Smedes, "is the painful feeling of being flawed humans . . . cracked vessels, wheels out of alignment. The heart of us slightly off center." [15] Shame tells us that as human beings, we all have limitations. Only God is perfect. We are, however, being perfected each day as we march on to perfection. Though we will never attain a total state of perfection in the sense of being without faults, defects, or being infallible, we are being perfected in our love for God and humanity, and in terms of our maturity as followers of Christ Jesus.

Shame leads us to hide behind a mask that covers our true self with a false self in order to conceal our guilt, limitations, inadequacy, and feelings of inferiority, not only from others but from ourselves. We are afraid that if our flaws are somehow revealed people will see us for who we really are. That could cause us humiliation and embarrassment. I agree with Bradshaw that, "A shame-based person will guard against exposing his inner self to others, but more significantly, he will guard against exposing himself to himself." [16]

In Matthew 19:16-22, a rich man approached Jesus with concerns about the kingdom of heaven. The rich man thought Jesus would justify him and perhaps praise him publicly for his good deeds and his flawless lifestyle. He asked Jesus, "Teacher, what good thing must I do to get eternal life?" (Matthew 19:16) Jesus' answer implied that he must obey all the commandments. The rich man boasted that he had practiced all the commandments since he was young. Jesus then told the man that if he wanted to enter the kingdom of heaven he should sell all of his possessions, distribute the proceeds among the poor, and then follow him. The man seems to have been so rich that he decided that such actions would be too hard, so he walked away feeling disappointed and perhaps embarrassed – and with a certain degree of shame and guilt. Jesus had revealed the man's true self to him and to others.

Did this man have a legitimate concern or could he have, perhaps, been a shame-based person seeking to be justified and affirmed by Jesus? It seems that Jesus saw through the man and knew the answer that he was looking for, but He was not about to give it to him. This man was fooling no one but himself. We can go on making people think we are somebody we are not, but in the process we risk having our true selves exposed.

When our identity is exposed and people see who we really are, they can become very disappointed with us. Our credibility then comes into question, adding to our emotional baggage, and as a result, our shame becomes greater. The sense of unworthiness can make us feel like an ostrich looking for a deep hole in the ground where we can bury our head. As the shame increases, anger and frustration can build up and place a heavy load on our shoulders. Metaphorically speaking, it can feel as if we were carrying an iron ball around our neck or a steel beam across our shoulders.

Guilt, according to Bradshaw, can be a toxic or healthy force in our lives. It can work in our conscience to let us know that we have gone against our values and beliefs. This kind of guilt is healthy. John Bradshaw comments that,

> Toxic shame needs to be sharply distinguished from guilt (guilt can be healthy or toxic). Healthy guilt is the emotional core of our conscience. It is the emotion that results from behaving in a manner contrary to our beliefs and values. [17] .

Healthy guilt can be a positive force. It can help get us back on track and prevent us from adding more shame to our emotional baggage. Guilt is like a voice telling our conscience, "See what you did? You went against all you stand for as a Christian and a minister. You just violated your core beliefs and values. You need to repent." Guilt, therefore, can be painful and can affect us internally until we recognize it and take a step toward repentance for our wrongdoing. Only then can we receive forgiveness. That forgiveness brings feelings of peace and freedom from guilt. Psalm 32, known as the "*ledavid Maskil*" Psalm of David, was written after David's transgression with Bathsheba and after obtaining forgiveness from God.

David had sinned against God when he went to bed with the wife of Uriah, one of his soldiers, while Uriah was fighting in the thick of battle. When David heard that Bathsheba had conceived a child, he sent for Uriah. In an attempt to cover up what he had done, David told Uriah to go home to his wife. He hoped that Uriah would go to bed with her so that the child in Bathsheba's womb could pass off as his. When Uriah refused to sleep with his wife, David sent him back to battle with a letter to Joab, instructing him to send Uriah to the front line where the fighting was fiercest, so that he could be killed. After the fight a report was sent to David informing him that Uriah was found dead. (2 Samuel 11:1-21) David had been guilty of three different sins: adultery (he slept with another man's wife which was contrary to the seventh commandment), deception (David wanted to trick Uriah into sleeping with Bathsheba so that he would think that the child was his), and homicide (a violation of the sixth commandment). Though David did not directly kill Uriah, he certainly plotted to have him sent to the thick of battle where he knew that Uriah would be killed. Since, David had been carrying the guilt associated with Uriah's death. In Psalm 32 David describes the pain produced by that guilt:

> Blessed is he whose transgressions are forgiven, whose sins are covered. Blessed is the man whose sin the Lord does not count against him and in whose spirit is no deceit. When I kept silent, my bones wasted away through my groaning all day long. For day and night, your hand was heavy upon me; my strength was sapped as in the heat of summer. Then I acknowledged my sin to you and did not cover up my iniquity. I said, "I will confess my transgression to the Lord," and you forgave the guilt of my sin. (Psalm 32:1-5)

Can you imagine the pain and agony that David was experiencing as he kept his sin from the world? David thought his transgression had been overlooked. Nevertheless, God sees all that we do and is always willing to forgive us if we confess and repent of all our sins. David had not just sinned against Uriah, he had ultimately sinned against God. All transgressions are committed against God, and then the person affected by the sinful act. It seems as though David had kept silent for some time, but a healthy guilt was like a voice inside his conscience calling to repentance saying, "Look what you have done. You slept with another man's wife. You have deceived him and then you send him back to battle with a letter declaring his own death sentence. You ought to be ashamed of yourself." The more David kept silent, the stronger the guilt and shame. He describes his guilt as emptiness, like a person totally dehydrated with his bones drying up. He describes feeling the weight of God's hand upon him sapping away all his strength, like the grass withering in the summer heat. In spite of the painful consequence of sin, David remained silent until the prophet Nathan added to his pain by denouncing his sin and admonishing him. David's admission of guilt and confession of sin prompted God to manifest his mercy. David received forgiveness and freedom from shame and guilt. God did forgive David, but if you read 2 Samuel 12:11-19, you can see that his sin had consequences for which David had a price to pay. The weight that guilt puts on our shoulders is like an alarm that serves as a constant reminder of our transgressions and need for repentance. We can say, therefore, that healthy guilt can be a positive thing.

Some Christians who have been brought up in strict Christian families often confess that they have experienced some degree of shame and guilt. The same is true (in some cases) with children who have been brought up in a pastoral family. There are so many norms, rules, and regulations that they must abide by. In addition, there are high expectations and higher standards set for these children that demand nothing less than perfection. These parents seem to overlook the fact that failure to live up to these demands could create harmful shame in their children. John Bradshaw comments:

> Perfectionism is a family system rule and is a core culprit in creating toxic shame. We will see it also in both the religious and cultural systems. Perfectionism denies healthy shame. It does so by assuming we can be perfect. Such assumption denies our finitude because it denies the fact that we are essentially limited. Perfectionism denies that we will make mistakes often and that it is natural to make mistakes. [18]

Though it is true that we, as believers in Christ, have been called to live a Christian lifestyle, in no way have we reached a state of perfection, nor will we attain such perfection during our lives. Even Paul the apostle, a man of great faith and one of the greatest contributors to the New Testament with his many epistles, did not think of himself as having attained a state of perfection. Paul writes to the congregation in Philippi:

> Not that I have already obtained all this, or have already been made perfect, but I press on, to take hold of that for which Christ Jesus took hold of me. Brothers, I do not consider myself yet to have taken hold of it. But one thing I do: Forgetting what is behind and straining toward what is ahead, I press on toward the goal to win the prize for which God has called me heavenward in Christ Jesus.
> (Philippians 3:12-14)

Paul believed that he was moving toward perfection, but he also understood that perfection (in the sense of being perfect, without fault or blameless) was a dynamic process that was not attainable in this world.

When parents want to force their children to be perfect by setting high standards and expectations for them, it can only lead to frustration, shame and guilt, especially when there are parents that are never satisfied with their children's accomplishments. Let's say that a child meets his/her parents' expectations, and instead of receiving a compliment from the parent they raise the bar to a higher standard. That is like telling them, "What you've done is okay, but not good enough. You can do better." As these children continue in their socialization process during their formative years, they will grow up believing that in order to please their parents they need to be perfect. When they realize that perfection is not within the realm of possibilities nor attainable in this life, chances are that they may become frustrated. No matter how hard they try, their parents will never reward or compliment them. This experience will become part of their emotional baggage as they reach adolescence and adulthood.

Erik Erikson, the American psychoanalyst who studied the influence of culture and society on child development, found a correlation between personality growth and parental and societal values. He affirmed in his concept of "identity crisis" the influence that parents and their social values have on the child. That influence shapes the growth identity in late adolescence. Erikson explains human development in eight psychosocial stages. In each stage, a child must go through a critical psychosocial conflict. Erikson says, "Every adult carries these conflicts with him in the recesses of his personality." [19] If a child is to advance successfully from one stage to another, that child needs to resolve each conflict at that particular stage. Failure to do that will cause the child to continue struggling with the conflicts into adolescence and adulthood. If left unresolved by adulthood, these conflicts can become part of a person's emotional baggage for the rest of their life. As a result, these conflicts can be triggered at any moment by association of an event or idea. In some cases it may result in shame and guilt or lead to embarrassment.

Emotional Baggage and Ministry

If we are to have emotionally healthy pastors and congregations, we need to work at dealing with our emotional baggage and solving the inner conflicts that we have been struggling with for years. This baggage can bring unhealthy shame, hurt our relationships, and hinder our ministries. Emotional baggage can be a harmful force for clergy, as it can become an obstacle that can preclude them from effectively carrying out their ministerial functions. Some (not all) clergy carry their emotional baggage like a backpack everywhere they go. This can and will affect their ministry in such a way that they become unstable, causing them to transfer out of one appointment and into another. In fact, some of these baggage-carrying pastors move from their local church on a yearly basis due to unresolved issues and their inability to deal with them. These changes in appointments could be spared if they would learn to deal with the contents of their emotional baggage before going to their new appointments.

Here are a few of the most common problems and personal issues that some clergy members might carry as part of their baggage.

Indebtedness

Financial indebtedness is one that some ministers face at the beginning of their career after graduating from seminary. Some clergy within the United Methodist Church are second-career persons. They leave a good-paying job or a professional career to answer God's call to ministry. They begin their preparation by enrolling in a Masters in Divinity (MDIV) program in seminary. During the course of their studies, they find themselves needing student loans in order to continue and complete their degree. Not too long after they graduate, they receive their first of many monthly statements from their student loan provider. When they get to their new appointment and take their first look at the pastor's compensation in the church budget, they realize that they are going to have to make adjustment in their personal budgets if they are going to make ends meet. After some time in their local churches some begin to get deeper in debt; and before long, they find themselves living from check-to-check. No sooner do they pay off one debt than they get into another.

Trying to get rid of debts can be difficult if one does not first admit that one has a problem. Some try to take the easy way out by borrowing from one source to pay another, but this only results in getting deeper into debt to the point that they walk into a point of no return. The more they try to get out of debt by these means, the harder it becomes. They may get so deep into debt that it could ultimately affect their ministry. When every attempt to work out their financial difficulty fails, they begin to have problems in their marriage and church relationships, which can and will affect their ministries. They try to keep their indebtedness from being publicly exposed, for fear that they would be labeled as irresponsible and a poor financial manager. Once discovered it could bring shame and guilt upon them.

When a person is about to be ordained as deacon or elder at the annual conference session of the United Methodist Church, he or she will appear before the clergy session for approval from all the elders and deacons in full connection. After a vote has been taken and the candidate has been accepted for ordination, the bishop examines him/her by asking a series of the Historic questions from Paragraph 330.d (1-19) of *The Book of Discipline of the United Methodist* (2008).These questions are presented to the candidate to "seek to interpret their spirit of intention." One of the questions that can put the person being ordained on the spot and make him/her feel uneasy is the one found in Paragraph 310.d (18), which reads, "Are you in debt as to embarrass you in your work?" [20] That question can put the ordinand in such an awkward position that he or she might hesitate to give an honest answer. However, we have no choice but to say the right thing, especially when we know that we are standing in the presence of God, the bishop, and the elders present at the annual conference session. No one likes to admit publicly that he or she is so indebted as to be embarrassed – more so if the individual is going to a pastoral appointment where he or she is responsible for the good stewardship of that ministry. That includes working with the church budget and the overall finances of the congregation. After all, how can one be a good steward of the finance and administration of the congregation when one cannot properly manage one's own household finances?

Some pastors who are heavily indebted may avoid preaching sermons on giving while leading their congregation through a stewardship campaign, because they themselves are poor managers of their personal finances. Some clergy may find it difficult to contribute with their tithes because they do not have much left after they pay their bills.

A pastor once invited me to preach on the first and last Sundays of a stewardship campaign. When I finished preaching the finance officer handed me a love-offering. After I thanked him, he said, "No, don't thank me. Thank my pastor for not wanting to preach and preferring that we pay someone else to do what he is supposed to do." When I asked him, "Oh, why is that?" he responded, "You can't preach what you don't practice."

Later on I found out that during the two years that pastor had served the congregation he was not contributing financially in any way. I also learned from one of the members that the pastor was very deep into debt. That is just one example of how indebtedness or poor financial management can impair a pastor's ability to fulfill his or her ministerial function responsibly and effectively. Eventually, the inability to deal with indebtedness may cause other emotional problems to surface. They may include anger, frustration, anxiety, or depression. To avoid getting to that point one needs to realize that he or she has a problem and needs help. The more unmanageable the situation becomes, the more one will become a walking time bomb ready to explode. Fortunately, there are a variety of ways to deal with this problem before it gets out of hand.

Working Toward a Solution to Indebtedness

The solution to indebtedness is not easy nor without cost. The first step is to realize that you have a problem and that the problem is affecting your family, congregational relationships, and your ministry.

Furthermore, the problem is not going to disappear without help. The good news is that there are public and private agencies where one can go for help. There may even be churches with programs that can assist you in your debt solution and budgeting.

Some people think an easy way to get out of debt is by filing bankruptcy. Many lawyers will be willing to help you in this process and perhaps get you on an affordable payment plan, in which you can send small amounts each month with little or no interest. You might even be able to have all your debts eliminated, depending on the chapter under which you file. The positive side of bankruptcy is that all debts are on hold and you are protected by the court against harassing phone calls from your creditors. The negative aspect of bankruptcy is that your file is sent to all three credit bureaus in the United States and will remain there for at least ten years. Worst of all is the humiliation of being publicly exposed. This is a bad witness to all your friends, church, and community members. After all, people do hold ministers to a higher standard. When they do not measure up to those standards, there is great disappointment and lack of trust among members of the congregation.

A better way to handle indebtedness is for the minister to go first before God to present the situation. Not that God is going to reach out with a magic wand and say, "Here, my child, your problem is now solved. You are completely out of debt." I wish it were that easy, but it is not. God provides human solutions for human problems. God is always willing to help, but God expects us to seek help from those human resources that He has provided. Presenting ourselves before God in prayer has more to do with asking God for some direction in solving the problem. To say that God cannot help us directly with whatever we need is to limit his power. God does what is in God's own will. Nonetheless, it is not ours to tell God how God should respond to our needs, or what course of action to take.

There are many financial planning resource agencies available to assist people with financial problems. There are financial advisers that can provide financial management counseling and a plan to get you back on track with your finances. But these services are not without cost. Perhaps some churches or social services have such programs. You may want to check on-line to see what is currently available in your area.

No matter where you go to solve your financial problems, you need to follow professional advice. Once out of debt, stay out of debt. This will help you to have a clear focus on ministry, healthy emotions, spiritual well-being – and one less emotional baggage to carry around.

Lack of Trust and Confidence

Trust and confidence are intimately related but have different meanings. Trust is defined as; "1*a* : assured reliance on the character, ability, strength, or truth of someone or something *b* : one in which confidence is placed . . .*

Trust can mean relying on a certain thing we believe has the ability to do something that we expect will be done on our behalf. Trust comes from *knowing* that we can rely on someone or something.

Confidence, on the other hand, is

> 1 *a*: a feeling or consciousness of one's powers or of reliance on one's circumstances <had perfect *confidence* in her ability to succeed> <met the risk with brash *confidence*> *b*: faith or belief that one will act in a right, proper, or effective way <have *confidence* in a leader> 2: the quality or state of being certain: CERTITUDE <they had every *confidence* of success>. *

It is a state-of-being and it comes from doing. When you are confident in someone, you trust that person's ability to do a specific thing that you know the person can do. You have probably seen the person in action, tested that person, and found him/her to be worthy of trust. Since you have placed your trust in their abilities, you are confident that he/she can assist you without failing. As human beings, we need someone we can trust and be confident that he/she will meet our spiritual, physical, and emotional needs. As Christians, we place our trust on God who provides love, care, and protection to God's children and gives us the ability to do the things that we cannot do for ourselves.

In many of his Psalms, David encourages believers to have trust and confidence in God. Throughout his life, David learned to trust in the Lord; when he found himself in times of trouble and in need of help, the mighty hand of God was upon him offering him comfort and strength. When David needed protection from his enemy, he trusted

---

* By permission, from *Merriam-Webster's Collegiate© Dictionary, 11th Edition* ©2013 by Merriam-Webster, Inc. (www.Merriam-Webster.com)

God with his life. He knew that God would be there for him. In times of persecution, David was confident that God would protect him from his enemy. No matter how great the danger or how difficult the situation, David was confident that God would come to his rescue if he would "let go and let God."

One of my favorite examples is Psalm 40, especially verses 1-4, in which David demonstrates his confidence in God in a very powerful way. The Psalm reads:

> I waited patiently for the Lord; he inclined to me and heard my cry. He lifted me out of the slimy pit, out of the mud and mire; he set my feet on a rock and gave me a firm place to stand. He put a new song in my mouth, a hymn of praise to our God. Many will see and fear and put their trust in the Lord. Blessed is the man who makes the LORD his trust . . . (Psalm 40:1-4)

The Psalmist does not mention what kind of a situation or danger David was going through when he wrote this Psalm. He may have been in the thick of battle, or facing persecution by his enemy. We have no clue as to what the situation might have been. However, we can imagine by the way he describes the situation, that he must have been desperate. David says he has fallen into a slimy pit (quicksand), and is trying very hard to save himself. If you are familiar with quicksand, you know that it will pull down any heavy object that falls into it. You do not realize the trap you are in until the quicksand starts pulling you down. Once in quicksand, it is very difficult to escape. One thing I learned about this slimy mire is that the harder you kick or try to pull your way out, the faster it will pull you down. Experts say that if you fall into a quicksand trap, the best thing to do is nothing. You just wait patiently while this wet sand slowly pulls you down and hope that someone might arrive in time to pull you out and take you to a safe place.

David probably knew about quicksand. He knew that the only way out was to trust in and wait patiently on God. Without a doubt, God would rescue him from this quagmire. David was confident in the Lord; he knew that God would never fail him. David's patience, confidence, and trust in God were amply rewarded when God saved him from danger and placed his feet on solid ground. In gratitude, David wrote this Psalm as a witness to God's unfailing love and care for all of

God's children. David trusted God regardless of the situation and declared a blessing on the man who places his trust and confidence in the Lord. David learned through experience, as a servant of God and as king of Israel, that our lives belong to God. We depend exclusively on God for strength, wisdom, and direction in life. David knew that, as king, the people would look to him for leadership and depend on him to meet their needs. But David knew he had human limitations. He knew there were things he could do on his own through his God-given abilities. For the more difficult tasks, he needed to have trust and confidence in the Lord.

That does not mean that we do not need to trust God for the simple things. It means that God has given us the ability to do certain things for others and ourselves within our human limitations, but in those circumstances where we are limited, God takes over and does for us what we cannot do for ourselves. David had an awareness of his God-given abilities, which made him feel very confident about himself. He knew he could do some things and do them well. They were things he had done routinely or had practiced for so long that they became natural to him. Plainly stated, David had a certain degree of self-confidence. He was sure he could do many things because he had knowledge, strength, wisdom, and abilities from God for those tasks. Nevertheless, his confidence in the Lord was always present in everything that he did.

Our greatest source of trust is God who has given us faith. Through that faith, we know God's unlimited power and ability to do all things in and through us. When we learn to trust God, God can use us in ways that we have never imagined.

Self-Confidence

In some Christian circles, the word *self-confidence* denotes a denial of faith, trust, and confidence in God. Some Christians I know claim that if you rely on your own knowledge, strengths, and abilities, you are arrogant and have no faith or trust in God. Nonetheless, I believe that God has given us certain gifts, talents, knowledge, and wisdom to use in ministry for the greater good and the benefit of the church and community. It is our God-given responsibility, as good stewards in ministry, to develop, strengthen, and use everything that God has given us to its full potential. I am confident that God can use any one of us at anytime and in any place – in spite of our human limitations – when we act responsibly. If we are self-confident, it is because we are certain that God has enough confidence in our abilities to let us minister to God's people. Furthermore, God has trusted us to do the things that God has empowered us to do. We, on the other hand, have trusted God to do the things we cannot do for ourselves.

However negative the concept of self-confidence may be for some Christians, it can be a very positive force in our lives and one that can influence others. People can tell when you are self-confident. When they perceive that you are self-confident they feel comfortable and safe around you – even in the most perilous situation. Self-confidence, like a pandemic, can spread from one person to the next and help calm any situation. Just appearing to be confident and being a non-anxious presence can help bring down the level of tension and anxiety in most situations.

We should always trust in our God-given abilities. They empower us to do the work of ministry that has been entrusted to us. Of course, we need to have confidence in the Lord for all things, especially those that transcend our human limitations. Only God can enable us to reach beyond those limits as God works in and through us for the benefit of God's kingdom.

Lack of Self–Confidence

Lack of self-confidence is one example of baggage commonly tucked away in a clergy's emotional backpack. Many people in the business world and in ministry fail to be successful in what they do because they lack confidence in their abilities. This lack of self-confidence can instill a pervasive sense of inadequacy in the individual that can keep them from moving up the ladder of success and rob them of many opportunities. Of course, others appear to be self-confident when they really are not. They do such a good job of hiding their fears and anxiety that people would think that they are self-confident. Still others are so obvious and transparent that people can almost see through them. Once such a person is exposed, people start losing trust and respect for him/her.

Gillian Butler and Tony Hope have designed a chart (see Figure 1) to show how "low self-confidence can affect the four aspects of life: your thinking, your feelings, your behavior, and your body." [21] The purpose of this chart is so that you can "Look at the box and think of your own level of confidence." They also suggest that you "adapt the list, if necessary, to fit your own experience." [22]

From this list, we can see that lack of self-confidence can affect us in many ways and make us feel very limited. Lack of self-confidence can produce self-doubt, denying ourselves the abilities that God has given us when we answered God's call to ministry. This effect also shows lack of confidence in God, through whom all things are possible.

Some of the effects of lack of self-confidence – Figure 1

Thinking
I can't.
That's too difficult.
I don't know how.
Maybe I won't be able to handle this.
It won't be good enough; someone else would do better.
I just can't decide what to do.

Feelings
Apprehension.
Anticipatory anxiety.
Worry, especially about forthcoming difficulties.
Frustration and anger with yourself.
Fear of the unknown or of new situations.
Resentment – it seems so easy for others.
Discouragement and feeling demoralized.

Behavior
More passive than active; keeping yourself in the background.
Finding it hard to make any suggestion, or putting yourself forward.

Prevaricating; being a slow starter.
Avoiding taking on anything new or making changes in your life.
Seeking help and advice even when you know the answer.
Hesitating – and repeatedly needing encouragement.
Taking a back sear.
Asking for reassurance.

Bodily signs of low confidence
Posture: tending to stoop, or retreating into yourself.
Not looking people in the eye.
Fumbling or fidgeting.
Feelings of tension and nervousness.
Sluggishness and lethargy.

Lack of self-confidence can deprive people of their initiative and limit their desire and ability to want to do anything. This effect can create a feeling of inadequacy, making us feel inferior to other people to the point that we think, "Why don't they ask somebody else to do it?" or "I wish I could be like him/her." People who think of themselves as inadequate tend to believe that other people have something they do not have; that others can do everything better than they can. These insecure people lack motivation. They might need encouragement to get started. Such people might find themselves in a state of ambivalence. They become incapable or perhaps unwilling to make decisions. This ambivalence could lead individuals into a cognitive- dissonant state. What they say and do is different from what their hearts feel. That is much like the people of Israel about whom Prophet Isaiah writes:

> The Lord says: These people come near me with their mouth and honor me with their lips, but their hearts are far from me. Their worship of me is made up only of rules taught by men. . . (Isaiah 29:13)

Figure 1 - From *Managing Your Mind: The Mental Fitness Guide* by Gillian Butler and Tony Hope reprinted by permission from Peters Fraser and Dunlop (www.petersfraserdunlop.com) on behalf of Gillian Butler.

The problem with cognitive-dissonant people is that they are not honest and up front. What they express verbally and through their actions is very different from what they feel in their hearts. You really do not know where these people are coming from, and you will never know where they stand on issues. That presents a problem of credibility, which is essential for ministry.

It is necessary to get past the shame that comes from having your true self exposed, and admit that you have a problem that needs to be dealt with. Of course, these emotional problems have no magic solutions. To start, I would recommend that you stop blaming and punishing yourself. Look at your strengths rather than your weaknesses. Look at yourself as a person of great worth, created in the image of God. See yourself neither as superior nor inferior to others. Accept that you are a human being with many limitations and imperfections. Do not be afraid to make mistakes, and do not be afraid to fail. If you fall, get back up and keep going. Most important of all, trust God and go before God's presence in prayer, asking God to help you deal with your lack of self-confidence. Self-confidence begins by having trust and confidence in the Lord and then having confidence in yourself. Be mindful that God has empowered you with the gifts, grace, and the ability to minister effectively to your church and community. It is encouraging to know that God will never fail or cause you to fall into shame, nor will God send you anywhere that God's grace will not accompany you. That is reason enough to feel confident in all that you do for God and God's people.

Low Self-Esteem

Self-confidence and self-esteem are two concepts closely related but with different meanings. Self-confidence has to do with having confidence in yourself and in your God-given abilities. Self-esteem has to do with self-confidence, self-image, and the way people perceive that others see them. Self-esteem also relates to self-worth, based on your self-evaluation. Self-esteem can be an emotional rollercoaster. At times people's self-esteem is so high that they feel great about themselves. They feel as if there is nothing in this world that they cannot do. At other times, self-esteem is so low that people feel low like a worm. They feel unworthy and think they have nothing to offer. They think the world looks down on them. Gillian Butler and Tony Hope observe:

> Self-esteem is a difficult concept. If it is high, we feel good about ourselves, and if it is low, we feel bad about ourselves. This much is straightforward. The higher the self-esteem, the more likely we are to achieve our potential and the lower the self-esteem, the more inhibited we will be. There is nothing so disabling as a sense of worthlessness. People who feel they are "worthless" or "do not count" also feel they have nothing to contribute. [23]

Low self-esteem denotes insecurity. It gives people the feeling of worthlessness. It makes them feel inadequate and inferior to others. David A. Seamands (1988), professor of pastoral ministries at Asbury Theological Seminary in Wilmore, Kentucky, considers low self-esteem one of Satan's deadliest weapons:

> An uneasy sense of self-condemnation hangs over many Christians like Los Angeles smog. They find themselves defeated by the most powerful psychological weapon that Satan uses against Christians. This weapon has the effectiveness of a deadly missile. Its name? Low self-esteem. . . . Satan's greatest psychological weapon is a gut-level feeling of inferiority, inadequacy and low self-worth." [24]

Nothing is worse or more denigrating than a person who has a low concept of him or herself and the resulting feelings of worthlessness and inferiority. Some people keep telling themselves that they are no good, that they do not have the ability to do the things that others do, that they are not good enough. Those people become so convinced of their worthlessness that they become stagnant. They feel they have nothing much to contribute to life, the church, or society. They limit themselves and feel inferior in comparison to others. People with low self-esteem tend to discount the good qualities they possess and to see the worse in themselves. They focus so much on their shortcomings that they think they have to walk on eggshells to avoid making mistakes. They fear criticism. These people feel that if they make mistakes and are criticized, they will end up being what they fear most – failures.

Overcoming Low Self-Esteem

If ministers and laypeople are to be effective in ministry, they need to realize that we are not perfect and that making mistakes is okay. Mistakes are part of a learning process. Therefore, mistakes do not matter. Everybody makes them. Butler and Hope agree that mistakes are inevitable and that errors are for learning:

> "The mistake made by confident people is to think that mistakes matter. If you tried every day for the next year to make a mistake that nobody had ever made before, you would most probably fail. What matters is not doing something 'wrong,' nor doing something 'badly,' but whether you can recognize the mistake and use it to try to set yourself on a better path next time. . . . Errors are for learning. Only those who have ceased to develop never take a wrong step. Mistakes are a source of information." [25]

Learning From Your Mistakes

Once we make a mistake, we cannot reverse what we have done. We need to accept our mistakes, take responsibilities for them, learn from them, and move forward. Dwelling on mistakes will contribute only to prolonging low self-esteem.

Learn to Handle Criticism

People with low self-esteem are over-sensitive to criticism. They care very much what people think about them. They are constantly judging and criticizing themselves. The last thing they need is for others to criticize them. When others criticize a mistake, learn to accept it. Remind yourself and others that you are human and that mistakes are common in all human beings. Look back at your mistake and ask yourself what you learned from the experience, then move on. Your mistakes should serve to make you better at what you are doing.

When I received my first appointment as pastor in a local church in 1984, I was compared constantly to previous pastors who had seminary training and more years of experience in ministry than I did. I took these remarks as criticism – not because I was incapable of the work but because I lacked the training and experience of my predecessor. However, I considered these criticisms as something positive, which would help me see my weaknesses and tell me what areas needed strengthening. When we learn to take criticism constructively – no matter how negative it may be – we begin to grow mentally, spiritually, and emotionally. When we feel offended by criticism and get defensive, we show our critics that we lack maturity, self-confidence, and willingness to learn from our mistakes. If we are to grow in all areas of our lives, we must accept criticism as a positive agent that could lead to transformation, growth, and development.

Have Self-Respect

If you want to gain respect, you have to start by respecting others as well as yourself. People with low self-esteem constantly belittle themselves. They describe themselves to others as worthless, incompetent, and incapable of doing anything. They tell themselves that they are not good enough to do things that others can do. Some will blame God for the way they feel about themselves. "I can't help it if God made me this way," they say. "I certainly got a dirty deal in life." God, however, is not to blame for the way we think or behave. That has more to do with how we process the experiences we accumulate in life from childhood to adulthood. Our experience during our formative years – good or bad, positive or negative – follows us for the rest of our lives and affects the way we think, feel, and act.

However, it is never too late to change our thoughts, feelings, and actions if we have the will to see ourselves differently. The way we think can change the way we feel, and the way we feel can change the way we act. The thing that we need to be mindful of is that God is willing and able to take you through whatever change you need to make in life. All you need to do is to trust in the one who will give you the strength to do it. Paul said, "I can do everything through him who gives me strength." (Philippians 4:13) If you believe this, you are well on your way to a transformative experience that can change your whole life.

Stress

Stress is a pervasive force; no living person can totally avoid it. We all live with a certain amount of stress. Therefore, we need to learn to deal with it before it reaches a level that produces high anxiety and depression.

Source of Stress

Many different sources, both internal and external, can produce stress. External sources are circumstances, events, or experiences outside of us and beyond our control. Examples of external sources can be trying to get to work on time and getting stuck in heavy traffic, driving down a lonely road late at night and getting a flat tire, or getting home and finding out that someone broke into your house and stole all the things that you worked hard for during your life. Internal stress factors include worrying excessively, being angry with someone, or feeling that something bad is going to happen.

Effects of Stress

Butler & Hope are in agreement about the difficulties of stress:

> One of the difficulties about stress is that it can work for you or against you, just like a car tire. When the pressure in the tire is right, you can drive smoothly along the road: if it is too low, you feel all the bumps and the controls feel sluggish. If it is too high, you bounce over the pot holes and easily swing out of control. [26]

I have experienced times when stress has worked for me. Other times it has gone the other way. When I was a student at Garrett Evangelical Theological Seminary in Evanston, Illinois, every one of my professors would pile a load of work on me as if their class was the only one I was attending. During midterms and finals each professor would assign a term paper. Some of these were due on the same day. I would calmly do the research and then – as I approached the due date and pressure began to build up – I would find myself looking at a blank screen, not knowing where to start. Nonetheless, building up a little stress sometimes had a positive effect on me. Pressure often made me productive and enabled me to finish the work on or before the deadline. Unfortunately, stress does not work that way for all people or in all situations. Stress has different effects, depending on the level. High levels of stress can have a negative effect that results in a lack of productivity and poor performance. Butler and Hope agree that, "For low levels of stress . . . increasing the stress can improve performance. High levels of stress, however, impede performance." [27]

Deadly Emotions

Stress is an unhealthy emotion. Like any emotion, it can be a powerful force within the human mind. Stress can affect the body and the soul. Jordan Rubin calls stress a deadly emotion that should be avoided. "Deadly emotions alter the chemistry of your body, and unchecked emotions can be a pervasive force in determining your daily behavior." [28] Stress can affect our physical, mental, and spiritual health. These three elements are intimately related and work as a system. Each component needs to work in harmony with the others. When any of these cease to function properly, the whole system is thrown off balance. When this happens, the system becomes dysfunctional.

Here are some effects that stress could have on our physical, emotional, and spiritual well-being:

Physical Health

Physical stress can interfere with normal bodily functions and change our lifestyles and eating habits in ways that can affect our health. In my personal life, I have experienced that stress had increased my appetite and craving for sweets. During my days as a seminarian, I would spend many hours in the library reading and doing research. Sometimes my stress level would rise to the point where I began to crave a snack. When this happened, I would make my way to the vending machine located in the hallway and get my daily supply of candy bars and various assortments of treats. Stress produced a strong craving for candy and other treats, which contributed to weight gain, and prompted the onset of Type II diabetes.

Stress can affect our thought process and our memory. Stress can bring about confusion and inability to make decisions. It can also produce anger, fear, and anxiety. When stress takes hold of us, we feel the effects on our mind and body. Stress affects how we think and feel. It can also affect us spiritually. When people experience stress, their mind and body feel tired and robbed of energy. They can also feel the tension on their shoulders and tightness in their chest. Stress can cause a person to lose focus on what is going on around them. Instead, they become so focused on themselves and their own situation that they close themselves off from the rest of the world. This physical and emotional separation can cause people to move away from their spiritual center and lose awareness of God's presence. The thing to do next is to let go of all your worries and trust God; for God is always present in our lives to help us in the midst of any situation, no matter how difficult.

Stress is not a respecter of persons. Everyone has experienced it in his or her life at one time or another. Some have experienced it at higher levels than others. No one is immune from this deadly emotional experience. Because of their position in the church, pastors are more prone to higher levels of stress than the people they serve. High demands and expectations are placed on pastors by their church, their family, and society. Many pastors work 50 to 60 hours or more a week. In addition to that, they have responsibilities as spouses and parents. Their weekly workload is so overwhelming that if they are not careful, they could be candidates for burnout. That is why pastors need to care for themselves while caring for the congregations – lest they become wounded healers.

Here are a few suggestions for pastors who find themselves stressed out and on the verge of burnout, from the long hours of work and high demands from the people they are called to serve.

Time Management

One of the most difficult tasks for pastors is time management. That can be difficult when you have so little time to do so many things in a day. Some pastors even wish that the day had more than 24 hours, in order to get everything done. I recommend that pastors start by setting priorities. They should reserve the first hour of the day for devotion and prayer. When we set time aside early in the morning to be in the presence of God, making devotion and prayer our first priority, God will take care of us for the rest of the day, giving us direction, guidance, and wisdom to make good use of our time and be effective in our ministry. God will also give us courage to meet our daily challenges. On the other hand, if we take off for work without presenting ourselves to God in devotion and prayer, we may find ourselves struggling through our day and time will seem to slip right through our fingers. We might also encounter many interruptions that will keep us from advancing in our work and meeting our deadlines. At the end of a long workday, we go home feeling tired and frustrated because we have accomplished very little. Therefore, it is important to make prayer and devotion the first thing we do each day.

Next, we need to prepare a work agenda or a "to do" list for each day. Bear in mind that many unforeseen events will interrupt our day. The key is not to do all the work on the agenda in one day, but to do the most important things first. It is not so important to do things right as it is to do the right things.

Finally, learn to manage your time. Do not let time manage you. Use your time wisely. Remember that the time you squander will not return. It becomes history. John Wesley was very mindful of time and considered it very valuable. One day at a pastor's retreat while preaching a sermon on stewardship, the preacher was trying to emphasize the importance of managing our time. To make his point he told the story about a man who approached John Wesley to ask if he could meet with him to share concerns he had about some theological issues. Mr. Wesley said he would meet the man the next evening after a prayer service, at a certain time and place. On the following day, he stood at the corner of the street where they were to have their meeting and waited for the man, who happened to be ten minutes late. When the man arrived Mr. Wesley said, "Young man, do you know that you just made me waste ten minutes of my time for the rest of my life?" Think about that. He lost ten minutes of his time for the rest of his life. He made a good point; time moves forward and cannot be rewound to make up for those lost and wasted minutes. The time we lose stays in the past never to return. It becomes history. That is why we need to use our time wisely and productively.

Time is very valuable and should not be misused or wasted by idling or procrastinating. Some people fall into a vicious cycle putting things off. An old saying goes, "Don't put off for tomorrow what you can do today." The problem with procrastinating is that the more you put the work on hold, the more work will pile up, putting you on hold. That can often cause frustration. When this happens, stress can develop and build up, and before you know it, you may find yourself in the verge of burning out.

Stress Reduction

You can reduce stress in a number of ways:

- Look for the warning signs of stress. Pay attention to your feelings, thoughts, and behavior.
- Do not over-commit or try to do more than you can handle.
- Be assertive. Say "no" when you mean no and "yes" when you mean yes.
- Manage your time wisely. Do not become a slave of time by letting time control you.
- Put your priorities in order. Do the first things first.
- Do not worry about what might happen. Cross that bridge when you get there.
- Remember, the important thing is not to do things right, but to do the right thing.
- Do what you can today, and remember that tomorrow is another day.
- Take time to relax and share with family and friends.
- Schedule some time on your calendar for vacation.
- Learn to delegate, not abdicate.
- Do not procrastinate. If you do, chances are things will never get done.
- Do not push yourself to the limit. When you need help, ask for it.
- It is not so important to be successful as it is to be effective.
- Accept responsibility for your mistakes.

Covenant Groups

Many clergy members provide pastoral care and counseling to the people in their church and community. They also try to help people solve their problems and help them find hope and meaning in their lives. Pastors, however, have no one to turn to for counseling or to help find solutions to their own problems. Pastors often become wounded healers in ministry, trying to heal others while they themselves need healing. Some pastors are reluctant to turn to their parishioners to find healing and comfort, thinking this could make them seem weak and vulnerable to the people they are supposed to minister to. Pastors are supposed to be spiritual leaders of their congregations; people expect them to be strong, with an unmovable faith and hermetically sealed emotions. To appear otherwise might appear as weakness or lack of trust and confidence in the Lord. These are only a few reasons why pastors dare not share their problems with lay member of their congregation.

To whom do pastors turn when they have problems? One person is their district superintendent – who is the extension of the bishop in the district. Among other things, superintendents are responsible for supervision of clergy members in their district. In that role, he or she is considered first among equals. By virtue of his appointment and call to ministry, he or she is, in a sense, pastor to the pastors in their district. Superintendents have a moral and ethical responsibility to maintain the confidentiality of information that clergy and laity in their district have placed in their trust. They also have an obligation to share any information with the bishop and cabinet, to which the superintendent is accountable. Some clergy members do not feel comfortable sharing their problems with their superintendent for fear it may be taken as a weakness or a sign that they are incapable of being effective in the local church. That, in turn, could lead to another appointment, which may be anything less than a promotion. In that case, to whom do pastors turn?

Clergy members are part of a covenant community of mutual trust and confidentiality, holding themselves accountable to one another. Clergy members experiencing difficult or stressful situations can seek help from one of their peers in this covenant group. Pastors can select a colleague with whom they are comfortable. They might look for someone who they can trust to keep the conversation under strict confidentiality. That person should be someone they know will listen, offer good advice, and provide support. Pastors should be very careful when selecting one of their peers. The person should be someone of the same sex in cases involving marital problems, especially if counseling is going to take multiple sessions. Same-sex counseling avoids emotional bonds that could complicate the situation. Remember, while Satan is on the loose, temptation is present. Temptation does not respect people or titles. Make sure you turn to someone who can help with your problem without creating a bigger one.

If you feel that there is no one among your peers that you can turn to, you can always consider going to a professional counselor for advice. Remember that professional counseling can be a lengthy and costly process. If you can afford it and are willing to pay, go for it. The important thing is that you can be restored from a wounded healer to a spiritually, emotionally, and physically healthy healer as you care for yourself before caring for others.

PART THREE:

PHYSICAL HEALTH

> *Do you not know that your body is a temple of the Holy Spirit, who is in you, whom you have received from God? You are not your own; you were bought at a price. Therefore honor God with your body.* (1 Corinthians 6:19-20)

Physical health, by medical standards, is measured by the general condition of the body at a given moment, especially the presence or absence of illnesses or physical impairments. Albeit, good health is not so much about the absence of a physical illness or limitations as it has to do with the way you look and feel. Jordan Rubin says:

> Good health is a lot more than the absence of disease in your life. Good health is waking up in the morning feeling rested and ready to attack the day. Good health is having the energy to keep up with those kids you're raising. Good health is having something left in your tank after you've put in a full day of work. Good health is thriving, not merely surviving. [29]

God's good intention is that we are healthy in every aspect of our lives. God makes us responsible for the way we take care of ourselves. A healthy body can increase our chances of living longer and having the energy necessary to carry out the mission God has called us to do. The human body is a gift from God. It belongs to God, not to us. The Apostle Paul regarded the body as something sacred. He makes it clear to us that we need to care for it properly so that God can use us for God's purpose, honor, and glory. God wants a healthy body in which God can be glorified. The apostle considers the body of a believer to be the temple of the Holy Spirit, who dwells in us. Our bodies, therefore, should have proper care. Paul said:

> Do you not know that your body is a temple of the Holy Spirit, who is in you, whom you have received from God? You are

> not your own; you were bought at a price. Therefore honor God with your body. (1 Corinthians 6:19-20)

Since our bodies belong to God, we need to be accountable to God not just for what we do with our bodies but also for how well we take care of them spiritually, emotionally, and physically. Rubin says:

> God owns our bodies, so we must honor God in the care of our bodies. Otherwise, we cannot continue God's work in the excellence of ascent. God intends to use my physical body through which the Holy Spirit can operate. . . . God needs our bodies to complete the mission of Jesus in the world. [30]

God wants to use us as God's servants. God wants us to be the vehicles by which God fulfills God's plan of salvation and God's mission in this world. God, through the Holy Spirit, wants to work in and through us to empower us for ministry and mission. God has called us to go to places we never expected to go, do things we never thought we would do, and minister to people we have never met, in places we have never been. We have many places to go and much work to do. Jesus told his disciples, "The harvest is plentiful but the workers are few. Ask the Lord of the harvest, therefore, to send out workers into his harvest field." (Matthew 9:35) The work is hard, with long hours and not much pay. The work can involve risk and sometimes danger. Nevertheless, the Lord of the harvest wants to send able bodies who are spiritually, emotionally, and physically healthy to take on this heavy yoke of ministry. Staying healthy is not as easy as some may think. It takes hard work and discipline, but in the end, it pays off. When we are healthy, we look younger, feel stronger, live longer, have more vitality, and become more fruitful.

The important thing is not just being healthy, but to stay healthy. To accomplish that, you have to live a proper lifestyle, get the right nourishment from eating proper foods, abstain from eating other foods or drinks that may contaminate your body, and avoid substances that might harm you with impurities or put your body at risk. Our bodies are as sacred and important to God as our mind and soul. We need to present them to God as a holy and living sacrifice, pleasing to God. Paul, being mindful of that truth, told the people in the congregation at Rome, "Therefore, I urge you brothers, in view of God's mercy, to offer your bodies as a living sacrifice, holy and pleasing to God–this is your spiritual act of worship." (Romans 12:1)

In the following pages, I discuss things we can do to keep our mind and body in good working condition each day.

Get a Good Night's Sleep

Slaughter highlights the importance of a good night's sleep as a way of renewing our body and mind:

> Sleep and relaxation are basic necessities of life in order to be alert and have the strength needed to carry you through the day. A good night's rest revitalizes tired bodies, gives us more energy, and helps us think more clearly throughout the day. [31]

Sleep deprivation is a common condition afflicting millions of American adults. This epidemic of sleeplessness can affect our bodies by making us feel tired and rundown the next morning. It produces stress, anxiety, and lack of emotional control. Lack of sleep weakens our immune systems. It lowers our defenses and makes us vulnerable to any harmful bacteria or infections that threaten our bodies. Any number of factors can cause sleep deprivation. Those include drinking caffeine or alcohol before going to bed, worrying excessively, and stress or excitement. Physical issues, such as hypertension, hypothyroid, or reaction to certain medications, can also keep us awake.

Not only does the lack of sleep affect our bodies. It can affect our minds as well. When we deprive our body of sleep, our thought processes can be impaired. Our ability to think and make decisions effectively is reduced. Our level of concentration and the brain's capacity to respond to certain situations declines. To function optimally during the day the body needs adequate sleep. The question is how much sleep is needed for the body to function properly. The need for rest varies from one person to another. The consensus is that most people need eight to nine hours of sleep each night. Yet some can function perfectly well on only three to four hours of sleep. Rubin, however, says our goal should be eight hours:

> Sleep experts say we have to shoot for the magic number of eight hours. Why eight hours? Because when people can control the amount of time they sleep, such as in a sleep

laboratory, they naturally sleep eight hours in a twenty-four-hour period.[32]

Here are some ways to get a good night's sleep:

- Go to bed early.
- Free you mind of all worries.
- Do not worry about the things you left undone at the office. Tomorrow is another day.
- Do not be anxious about tomorrow. Live day-to-day.
- Learn to relax the body.

Rest and Relaxation

Our bodies can take a lot of physical and mental abuse, but we cannot function properly without a break when overloaded. We need to take some time off to rest from the busy and stressful workweek. The body needs to rest so it can restore the energy that it has expended during the week.

Most pastors take Fridays off as their day of rest. Nevertheless, they often use that time to work on their sermons. Others prefer to take Mondays off while their spouse is working and the kids are in school. That gives the pastor very little or no time during the week to share with their family. Some pastors use their time off to work around the house or prepare for church events, Bible study, or their next sermon – in case an emergency arises that might take their preparation time away later in the week. Before they know it, the week is gone, and they have not had the opportunity to spend time with the family or take time to rest their tired bodies and minds. This can result in poor physical and emotional well-being and may also create problems in their family relationships.

Pastors need to be mindful of the fact that they have a family who needs them. They need to schedule some quality time with them. Pastors also need to take time for rest and relaxation so that they can renew both physically and spiritually. Depriving themselves of rest can be a harmful thing. Our bodies, our families, and our time are all gifts from God. We need to care for ourselves in order to care for others. Therefore, pastors need to learn to delegate tasks to church leaders. They can take care of church business while the pastor takes time to relax mentally and physically. Do not worry about the work you leave behind when you take a day off or go on vacation. It will be there when you get back. Take care of it then. While on vacation, try, as much as possible, to get away from home or the work environment. Leave your house and office. Otherwise, you may be tempted to go to work.

Even the heart needs time for relaxation to perform properly. It needs to take time for a cardiac cycle called "absolute refractory period." The refractory period, according to Rubin, is a medical term that describes a period when the "heart cannot beat." Rubin says:

> After each contraction of the heart, known as the systole, there is a time of relaxation from the work that has been done. In medical terms, we call this the absolute refractory period – a time in the cardiac cycle when the heart cannot beat. During this period of relaxation, known as the diastole, the heart not only recovers, but it also refills with blood."[33]

The absolute refractory period can serve as a metaphor for the body's need for rest and relaxation. As our heart needs to rest during the cardiac cycle, our bodies need to rest during the 24-hour day cycle. Another example of our body's need for rest is found in Genesis 2:2-3:

> By the seventh day, God had finished the work he had been doing; so on the seventh day he rested from all his work. And God blessed the seventh day and made it holy, on it he rested from all the work of creating that he had done.

In Genesis 1, God begins God's work of creation. The task took six days. On that sixth day, God finalized God's mighty work by creating man and woman. On the seventh day, God rested from God's labor and sanctified that day. In Exodus, God handed to Moses a tablet with ten commandments. One was to honor the Sabbath:

> Remember the Sabbath day by keeping it holy. Six days you shall labor and do all your work, but the seventh day is a Sabbath to the Lord your God. On it, you shall not do any work . . . for in six days, God made the heavens and the

> earth, the sea, and all that is in them, but he rested on the seventh day. Therefore, the LORD blessed the Sabbath day and made it holy. (Exodus, 20:8-11)

God not only created and rested on the seventh day, but also charged us to keep the Sabbath as a day of rest, by including it as one of the Ten Commandments. For this reason, it is important that clergy take one day out of the week from their busy schedule for rest and relaxation from their labors. Some people, including clergy members, are addicted to their work. They take very little time for their families or themselves. They work long hours and spend little time at home. They often take their work home, get a few hours of sleep, and go off to work early the next morning. Some even confess that they get up in the middle of the night to catch up on some of their work. Their whole life seems to revolve around nothing but work. Rest and relaxation have been excluded from their vocabulary.

It is good to love and value your work as something precious given to us by God. It is a means of sustaining our families and ourselves. But when work becomes the most important thing in our lives – above family, friends, and social interactions – that is a very critical issue. People who fall under this category are known as workaholics. There is a difference between a hard worker and a workaholic, however, and we must not confuse one with the other. Hard workers are intentional about what they do. They will concentrate on their work and expend time, energy and effort during their normal work hours to get the work done. Once they have finished their work for the day, they go home to have time with their family and/or friends. They know how to separate their work from their personal time. Workaholics, on the other hand, do not have a life apart from their work. Work is the only thing they live for, and practically the only thing they think about. Work is the only satisfaction they get in life.

Like alcoholism or any other kind of addictions, work-a-holism can be serious and can destroy families or individuals. It can bring about serious stress-related health problems that can affect people physically, emotionally, and spiritually. When this happens, it is time to seek help before there is burnout or any emotional damage that this may cause. In many cases these stress-related problems, if prolonged, could lead to deadly emotions (already mentioned in Part Three). These could result in anger and hostility which can affect us physically, emotionally and (perhaps) spiritually.

Hypertension and Diabetes

Two common diseases that can result by not taking care of ourselves are hypertension and diabetes. Excessive stress and poor lifestyle choices can affect and complicate both conditions.

Hypertension

Hypertension (high blood pressure) is a blood pressure reading that is persistently at or above 140/90. The systolic pressure measures the pressure in the blood stream during the normal rhythmic contraction of the heart, as the blood is being forced through the aorta and the pulmonary artery. A blood pressure reading of 120 (systole) over 80 (diastole) would be considered normal by most physicians. Hypertension is often called the "silent killer." That's because, in most cases, it has no noticeable symptoms. You could, therefore, have hypertension and not know it until you go to the doctor for a check-up. If left untreated, hypertension could have serious consequences.

Causes of hypertension

The major cause of hypertension is unknown, but one thing we do know is that tension and stress can/may lead to this condition. One popular belief is that genetics can lead to hypertension. However, specific genes have not been identified. Some sustain the belief that if one parent has hypertension, the children are likely to have high blood pressure as well. Smoking, drinking, excessive sodium, obesity, and lack of exercise can contribute to increased blood pressure.

No matter what may be the cause of hypertension, health authorities agree it can be a health risk. However, if the condition is diagnosed early it can be controlled. To detect hypertension at an early stage you must have your blood pressure checked. Hypertension is silent and you may have it without knowing it. If you think that you might be at risk you should schedule an appointment with a doctor to have your blood pressure checked. Once hypertension has been diagnosed, the doctor can treat it with medication or by recommending a program of diet, exercise, and weight loss. The doctor may also recommend eliminating salt from your diet.

Diabetes

Equally as dangerous as hypertension is diabetes mellitus (sugar diabetes). Diabetes is the inability of the pancreas to produce sufficient insulin to reduce blood sugar content (glucose), or the patient may be insulin resistant. As glucose travels throughout the body without being absorbed, sugar concentration accumulates in the blood. The kidneys eventually filter the sugar from the blood and into the urine, which carries excess blood sugar from the body. Diabetes comes in two major forms: Type I and Type II. Type I (insulin-dependent) diabetes can develop in very small children. Ford-Martin and Blumer have this to say about this type diabetes:

> Type 1 diabetes, sometimes called juvenile diabetes, childhood diabetes, or insulin dependent diabetes mellitus (IDDM), occurs when 90 percent or more of the pancreatic beta cells have been destroyed, usually by an autoimmune process that impels the body to attack itself. [34]

Type I diabetes is treated with insulin. The diabetic must inject insulin to regulate the blood sugar levels. In addition, the treatment requires exercise and a special diet. Type II diabetes appears most often in people over 40. Again, according to Ford-Martin and Blumer:

> Type 2 diabetes, the most common type of diabetes is also one of the most prevalent chronic diseases around. More than 150 million people suffer from this disease; the International Diabetes Federation projects that this population will double globally by the year 2025. [35]

This diabetes is non-insulin dependent. The pancreas can produce sufficient insulin, but the body cannot absorb the insulin properly. Symptoms of Type II diabetes can begin so gradually that a person may not know that he or she has it. However, there are certain symptoms that can serve as a warning to us about the possibility of diabetes. It is not unusual for Type II diabetes to be detected while a patient is seeing a doctor about another health concern.

Causes for diabetes

Although causes of diabetes are unclear, at least three factors are known to contribute to the development of diabetes: environment, heredity, and obesity.

Environmental Factors

Alterman and Kullman make the case that a person's environment, which includes the lifestyle and behaviors can play a significant role in obesity. [36] And obesity, as many researchers agree, can be associated with diabetes.

Hereditary Factors

In Type II diabetes, age, obesity, and family history play an important role. Research shows that some people with diabetes have common genetic markers. Chassnoff, Ellis, and Fainman note, "Research shows that people who have Type II diabetes in their families have a greater tendency to acquire the condition." [37]

How is diabetes treated?

Diabetes has no known cure. It can, however, be controlled. Type I diabetes is treated with insulin, exercise, and diet. Adherence to the prescribed diet is an important aspect of controlling elevated blood sugar. Weight reduction and exercise are important treatments because they increase the body's sensitivity to insulin. This helps control blood sugar levels. The initial treatment for Type II diabetes is diet, exercise, and weight reduction. If that does not work, oral medication can be added. In most cases, where oral medications fail to control high levels of blood sugar, an insulin injection is necessary.

Obesity Crisis

Obesity contributes to both hypertension and Type II diabetes. Obesity is one of the biggest health problems in America today. The condition affects a large proportion of the total U.S. population. And obesity is not just an adult thing. The problem affects many children. A study by Paula Ford-Martin and Ian Blumer shows that,

> An estimated 5.3 million, or 12.5 percent, of Americans between six and seventeen are obese. Childhood obesity has led to an alarming increase in Type 2 diabetes, once considered an "adult–only" disease, and can lead to a variety of other weight-related medical problems later in life. [38]

The latest data from the World Health Organization global looks at obesity in children. "The statistics," said Dr. Manny Alvarez, health adviser for Fox News, "predicted that by 2010 a lot of children on this planet were going to be overweight." [39] That is completely different from past generations. The current prevalence of obesity among children is very troubling. If these statistics do not change, this generation of children is going to be dealing with higher numbers of Type II diabetes and hypertension. This is going to have a tremendous impact on their life spans. The number of obese people in the United States had rapidly increased in the past decade. "According to a study performed by the Archives of Internal Medicine, the ranks of extremely obese grew from one in two thousand in 1996 to one in four hundred in 2000." [40] Sad to say, the number of children with Type II diabetes is increasing rapidly along with the rising obesity rates.

Defining Obesity

So, how do we define obesity? Moreover, how is being obese different from being overweight? Alterman and Kullman explain:

> To be obese means to be considerably overweight . . . Overweight refers to body weight in excess of the normal range that includes all tissues-muscles, bones, and fat – as well as water. Obesity refers specifically to having excess body fat.[41]

There is general agreement among doctors, "that men with more than 25 percent body fat and women with more than 30 percent body fat are obese." [42]

Alterman and Kullman suggest two simple, but less reliable, methods for estimating body fat to determine if a person is overweight. "One is to measure skinfold thickness with a special type of caliper in several parts of the body. The second involves sending a harmless electric current through a person's body (bio-electric impedance analysis)." [43] This can be done through the use of an electronic machine, such as the ones used by trainers in a gym. Doctors, however, prefer to use body mass index (BMI). This measurement takes into account a person's weight and height. Doctors often use BMI weight-for-height tables to determine if the person has a weight problem. These charts make calculation easy.

On the following page is a BMI Chart. The vertical rows show weight measured in pounds. The horizontal columns show height measured in feet and inches. The number where height and weight columns intersect is the BMI. The formula for calculating the index, as Alterman and Kullman suggest, is BMI = km/m^2. In other words, "BMI equals a persons weight in kilograms divided by the height in meters squared." [44] Therefore, if you want to find the BMI for a person 35 or older, look at the chart. If the number is more than 27, the person is considered obese. For people 34 or younger, according to Alterman and Kullman, "a BMI of 25 or more indicates obesity." [45]

Causes for Obesity

We know one of the ways to become overweight is to overeat – ingesting more calories than your body can burn. Lack of physical activity and exercise contribute to obesity. In many cases, a persons' eating pattern, as well as his or her eating habits and preferences, can also be a contributing factor toward obesity. "Skipping and consuming most of the daily caloric intake with the evening meal can lead to obesity." [46] In some cases, physical and psychological disorders could lead to overeating and obesity. However, these are not the only causes. "Evidence suggests that obesity often has more than one cause. Genetic, environmental, psychological, and other factors all may play a part." [47]

Figure 2 - BODY MASS INDEX (BMI), kg/m²						
	-------------------- Height (feet, inches) --------------------					
Wt (lbs)	5'0"	5'3"	5'6"	5'9"	6'0"	6'3
140 lbs	27	25	23	21	19	18
150 lbs	29	27	24	22	20	19
160 lbs	31	28	26	24	22	20
170 lbs	33	30	28	25	23	21
180 lbs	35	32	29	27	25	23
190 lbs	37	34	31	28	26	24
200 lbs	39	36	32	30	27	25
210 lbs	41	37	34	31	29	26
220 lbs	43	39	36	33	30	28
230 lbs	45	41	37	34	31	29
240 lbs	47	43	39	36	33	30
250 lbs	49	44	40	37	34	31

Genetic Factors

Some people have a natural tendency to be obese because of their genetic predisposition. "Obesity tends to run in families suggesting that it may have a genetic cause." [48] We see both overweight parents and children. That could signal a hereditary factor. The good news is that even if you have a genetic predisposition to be overweight, you can do many things to control your weight.

Environmental Factors

"Although genes play an important role in some cases of obesity, a person's surroundings have effects. Environment includes lifestyle behaviors, such as what a person eats and how active he or she is." [49] Saudek, Rubin, and Shump agree that unless a person modifies his or her behavior, they will not lose weight. [50]

Figure 2 By permission from: Alterman, Seymour L., and Kullman, Donald A. *Diabetes: Prevention, Control, and Cure.* New York : Ballantine Books, 2004

One way to modify behavior is to recognize the need for change and then initiate a process to bring that change about gradually. For instance, instead of serving yourself a large portion of food, try dishing out a third less of that portion. Rather than filling your mouth and swallowing your food without chewing it properly, take small bites. Concentrate on each bite, and try to savor the flavor as you chew. Try pausing a few seconds between bites. Instead of drinking a soda, drink a glass of iced tea or water. Do not eat to feel full. Eat to feel satisfied. As you change your eating habits, you will get used to eating less. "The theory is that if you can recognize and pinpoint a specific moment when your behavior needs changing and can work out a way to keep bringing that need for change to the front of your mind, you can successfully modify behavior." [51]

Psychological Factors

Alterman and Kullman believe that there may be psychological factors involved in obesity. They suggest that, "Psychological factors also may influence eating habits. Many people eat in response to negative emotions such as boredom, sadness, or anger." [52] Eating is used as an outlet. They constantly put food into their mouths to get the sensation of feeling full. They want to substitute that feeling for other emotions. Emotional eaters consume more calories than they can burn and begin to store the excess fat. When that happens, it is time for them to admit that they have a problem and need to seek help. In many cases, they may need professional counseling to help them deal with the problems causing the eating disorder. Once underlying problems are addressed, the person should get into a behavior modification program that can help them make changes in their lifestyle. In so doing, they may be able to lose weight and keep it off.

Risks of Obesity

There was a time when being heavy was thought to be a sign of health. Chubby babies were seen as cute with their puffy, red, rosy cheeks, and big arms and legs. A woman was considered sexy if she had a little extra weight on her body. However, what was once considered healthy and sexy is totally opposite to current views. That is especially true since medical research has linked obesity to poor health. Saudek, Rubin, and Shump mention that Type II diabetes and hypertension are associated with obesity:

> Why do we talk so much about high blood pressure and diabetes? Because any way you look at it, they are closely related. One reason for this is that Type II diabetes is associated with being overweight, and so is high blood pressure. [53]

Obesity and Hypertension

Health professionals had focused on hereditary factors that put health at risk. With the current epidemic of obesity, they are looking at excess weight as one of the biggest risk factor. Obesity is common among hypertensive patients. In fact, obesity may be what determines the increased incidence of high blood pressure with age. Obesity can contribute to hypertension and "makes control of high blood pressure more difficult." [54] For one thing, obesity leads to greater blood output. The heart must pump more blood to supply the excess tissue. The increased cardiac output can raise blood pressure. In addition, insulin resistance occurs more frequently in the obese. "It has been theorized that the hypertension may, in some way, be related to the insulin resistance that is found not only in diabetes, but also in obesity." [55]

Obesity and Type II Diabetes

Just as high blood pressure and being overweight are closely associated, medical research has found a link between Type II diabetes and obesity. In an article for *Diabetes Spectrum* titled, Obesity and Type 2 Diabetes: The Twin Epidemic: Preface, Sonia Caprio, MD and Guest Editor says:

> The recent increase in the prevalence of obesity is closely paralleled by the increase in the prevalence of diabetes. Indeed, this new unprecedented phenomenon has been referred to as "diabesity." There is a clear strong relationship between obesity and the risk for diabetes. [56]

Carrying extra body weight and body fat contribute to the development of Type II diabetes. Being overweight puts people at greater risk of developing Type II diabetes than those individuals who are not obese. Excess weight puts added pressure on the body's ability to control blood sugar using insulin. That makes diabetes much more likely.

Treating Diabetes and Hypertension

The good news is that hypertension and Type II diabetes are treatable and preventable. Research has found that even small weight loss can prevent or delay the development of Type II diabetes and hypertension. You can control your blood sugar and your overall health by exercising regularly and changing your lifestyle.

Weight Reduction as Treatment

Weight loss is very important in treating problems related to obesity. Blood pressure and the risk of developing diabetes can be decreased significantly by losing weight. According to Saudek, Rubin, and Shump, if a diabetic can lose some weight, "the insulin output of the pancreas may very well be sufficient, and the person may no longer have diabetes." [57] I certainly agree with that statement in that losing weight could help lower the blood sugar in diabetics. I remember a time when I was weighing 215 pounds. I had difficulty keeping my blood sugar at its normal range. There were times when my glucose levels would go up to 250 and above. Every morning and evening I would take 35 units of insulin along with one metformin 1000mg and glyburide 10mg, yet I still could not keep my sugar level low. My doctor told me that it was possible that I had become insulin-resistant due to my obesity. He recommended that I get into a diet and exercise program in order to lose weight and replace the fat with muscles. This would make my insulin more productive. For the longest time I tried losing weight by eliminating breakfast and eating a light lunch, but in the evening, I would make up for what I had not eaten for breakfast or lunch. I realized then that I had to make changes in my life, so I decided to get into a disciplined regimen of diet and exercise.

The following week I made an appointment with the hospital dietician and she signed me up for a class on nutrition. Next, I signed up for membership at Gold's Gym. On the following day, I got started with my diet and exercise program. During my first week, I felt disappointed because I had not noticed any weight loss. The second week I felt discouraged and did not think it was going to work. However, on the third week I started to notice that my pants were fitting a little loose. I noticed that I was starting to lose some weight. That is when I began feeling motivated and feeling good about myself. This was an incentive for me to continue what I was doing. After a few months of exercise, I dropped from 215 pounds to 200 pounds. Then to 185 pounds, and now I am at 175 pounds and able to maintain. The good news is that not only did I go down in my weight, but also I was able to better control my diabetes and blood pressure with much less medication, a proper diet, and daily exercise. It was hard at first, but I have been able to adapt. I am still a diabetic and have to take medications (a very small amount), but my diabetes and hypertension are under control and my energy level is high. This is living proof that losing weight can significantly lower both your blood sugar and blood pressure. This would not have happened if I had not decided to lose weight.

Losing weight, however, is not an easy thing. It takes hard work, discipline, changes in lifestyle, and attitude. It also means that we need to acquire new eating habits if we are to live a healthy life. These are some new eating habits you should learn:

- Choose meals that are lower in fat.
- Do not eat when you are not hungry.
- Eat three meals a day. Do not skip a meal.
- Eat a good nutritious breakfast.
- Drink water instead of soda.
- Eat baked, broiled, roasted, or grilled rather than fried foods.
- Eat moderate portions of nutritious foods.
- Take a 15-minute walk after eating.

Most of all, remember that, "If you consume 500 calories a day less than your requirement, you'll lose a pound a week." [58] Changing your eating habits and dieting are not enough to lose weight and maintain a healthy body. You need to exercise to burn calories and tone your muscles. Once you decide to lose weight, I would recommend that you not think it over twice. Make a commitment to start an exercise program and receive the long-term benefits that increased activity will bring.

Exercise Program

A regular exercise program may help lower blood pressure and blood sugar over the long term. For example, simple exercise, such as walking, jogging, swimming, or bicycling, will help lower your blood pressure and glucose level significantly. All it takes is about 30 to 45 minutes a day. You will begin to see results immediately. There seems to be a correlation between the amount of exercise and the degree to which the blood pressure and blood sugar levels are lowered. Therefore, the more you exercise and the more intense your physical activity, the more you will be able lower your blood pressure and blood sugar. Exercise will not only serve as a treatment for obesity-related conditions. It will make you feel better and look good as those extra pounds melt away. However, there are some things you must consider before you begin your exercise program:

- Consult your health provider before starting.
- If you have to lose weight, do it slowly.
- Determine your heart rate at rest and during activity to see the intensity of your exercise.
- Always warm up before beginning a workout. Do muscle stretches before you start workout to avoid pulling a muscle.
- Always cool down after exercise.
- Start at a moderate pace. Do not try to do too much too soon.

Not too many people find exercise enjoyable. Some find it boring, time consuming, strenuous, and painful. They come up with many excuses for avoiding it. Many people have a hard time setting aside time for exercise. Remember that a little exercise is better than no exercise at all. You have to plan for it.

You can get started with your exercise program several ways. Saudek, Rubin, and Shump suggest that you set goals to avoid pitfalls. They further suggest that you draft a written exercise contract with yourself.[59] This contract commits you in writing to doing the exercise at a scheduled time and holds you accountable for accomplishing your program goals and objectives. The suggested contract looks like this:

EXERCISE CONTRACT
Exercise goal for week of July 3
Activity: Walking 12 blocks in 30 min.
Exercise goal for week of July 10
Activity: Walking 15 blocks in 35 min.
Exercise goal for week of July 17
Activity: Walking 15 blocks in 30 min.[60]

One important thing in an exercise program is the motivation level of the person. People are motivated by knowing what the results of their hard work will be. They increase their motivation when they see those results. The Energy Expenditure Chart on Figure 3 will let you know how many calories you burn with each exercise. It will also help you select a proper exercise program, set and reach your goals, motivate you, and hold you accountable.

Choosing Your Exercise Program

In choosing your exercise program your first question might be, "How much is membership to a health and fitness club going to cost me?" The truth is that when it comes to your health, money should not be an object. Remember that when you start your exercise program, you are investing both your time and money to your good health. Many gyms in your area are very affordable and provide trainers. They will help you select a proper exercise program, set your goals, motivate you, and hold you accountable.

Getting Started

Before you start your exercise program, you need to set some goals. For example, you need to know how much weight you want to lose and how long it will take you to lose it. Determine how much excess body fat you have. You can do this by using the BMI chart on page 76. Look at the number where your height and weight columns intersect. Anything above 27 is considered obese. Do not try to do too much too soon. The slower you lose weight, the easier it will be to keep it off. The important thing to remember is that diet and exercise go hand and hand. Just because you are dieting and exercising does not give you permission to throw yourself on the smorgasbord.

Figure 3 - Calorie Expenditure Chart

Activity/Exercise	Calories per Minute
Playing golf (carrying clubs)	6-7
Playing golf (golf cart	3-3.5
Swimming	5-6
Skating	8-9
Rowing	11-12
Dancing (moderate)	4-5
Dancing (aerobic)	10-11
Cycling	6-10
Standing	2-2.5
Sitting	1-1.5
Sleeping	1-1.5
Gardening	6-7
Walking at 3 miles per hour	4-5
Walking at 4 miles per hour	6
Jogging	10-12
Running	14-16
Lifting Weights	9-10
Playing Basketball	11-12
Mopping	3.5- 4
Vacuuming	3.5- 4

Figure 3 – By the author

Whether you are going to train in a gym or at home, you must first consult with your physician. He or she will advise you on the level and intensity of the exercise. Because a lot of the fat-burning exercise will involve cardiovascular workout, which accelerates your heart rate, you need to know if your heart can handle the stress. You must determine your maximum heart rate.

You must determine your maximum heart rate by either consulting with a physician or professional certified trainer who can calculate that for you. One formula that was taught to me when I was starting my exercise program in the gym was, to subtract your age from your weight and the difference between the two would be your (mhr) maximum heart rate. For example; a person 52 years of age and weighing 220 lbs. would need to use the following formula to find his/her maximum heart rate: 220 – 52 = 168 (mhr). Let's say you want to exercise at a 50% intensity. You would have to multiply your (mhr) by the percentage of your intensity. The formula would look something like this: 168 (mhr) x 50% (intensity) = 84 (thr). This would be your target heart rate at a low range. For a higher range, multiply by a higher intensity. For example, 168 x 70% = 118 (thr).

Therefore, target heart rates between 84 and 118 will make exercise safe and effective. You should test your heart rate before and during your workout. Put your palm face up and place the middle and index finger of your other hand on the artery that is in line with your thumb. Count the beats for 30 seconds. Multiply the number of beats by two. Alternatively, you can count for six seconds and multiply by 10. The total number of beats is the heart rate. You can also check your pulse by placing your index and middle finger on the side of your neck near the larynx and count the number of beats just as you would on your wrist. While exercising you should check your pulse at least every 10 minutes.

Warm–Up

You should never start to exercise without first warming up for at least five minutes and doing some muscle stretches. If you fail to do that, you could pull a muscle, or you could feel pain on the following day. If you have an exercise bicycle or treadmill, use it for at least six minutes. Do at least 90 seconds at a moderate pace. Then work your way up to a fast pace for the next 4½ minutes. If you do not have a treadmill or bicycle, walk for about two minutes and then jog for about four minutes. If you are indoors, you can run in place. After warming up check your pulse. Your heart rate should be at the minimum target heart rate for starting your exercise routine.

Muscle Stretch Routine

Now you are ready for some muscle stretches. They will protect you from pulling a muscle during exercise and soreness later. Be sure to stretch every muscle group, concentrating on upper and lower extremities, back, legs, chest, arms, shoulders, and sides. Do not overstretch your muscles to the point that they begin to hurt. There can be gain without pain. The key is to stretch until you can feel a slight tension on the particular area you are working on. On the following pages are some suggested warm-up exercises.

Calf Stretch

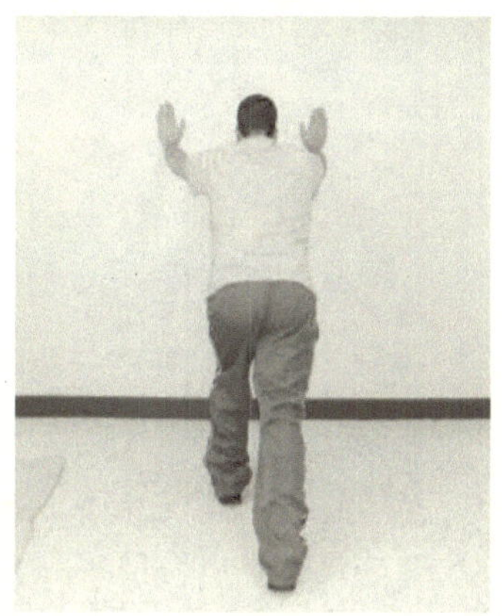
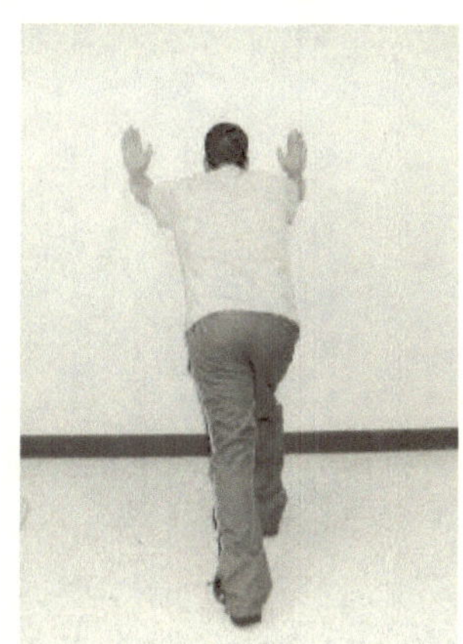

With your arms stretched parallel to the floor, put palms flat against the wall. Extend your right leg as far back as possible. Bring your left leg forward, and bend your left knee. Keep both feet flat on the floor, and lean forward until you feel tightness on your calf. Switch legs, and repeat exercise.

Leg Stretch

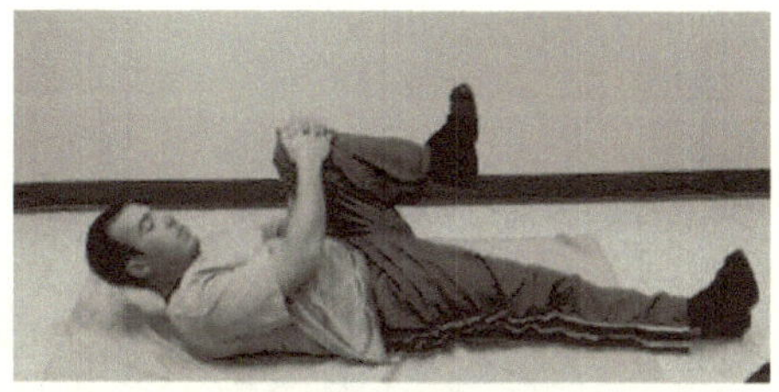
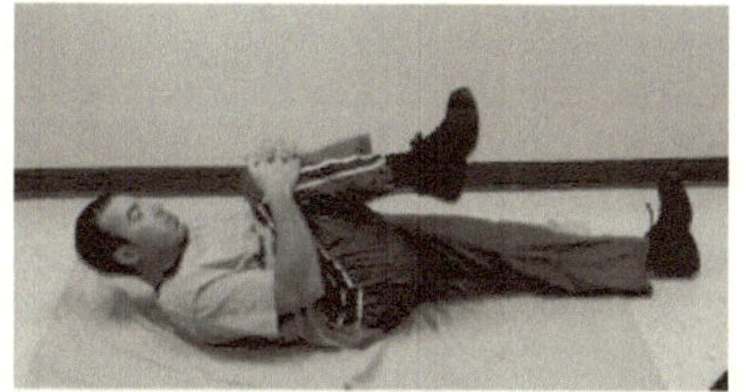

Lie flat on your back. Bend your left leg while stretching your right leg outward. Place both hands on your right knee, and bring your leg as close as possible to your chest for about five seconds. Switch legs, and repeat exercise. Do 15 repetitions.

Shoulder Stretch

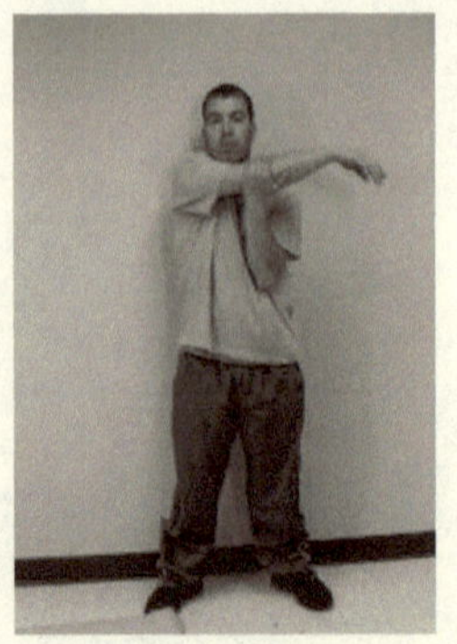
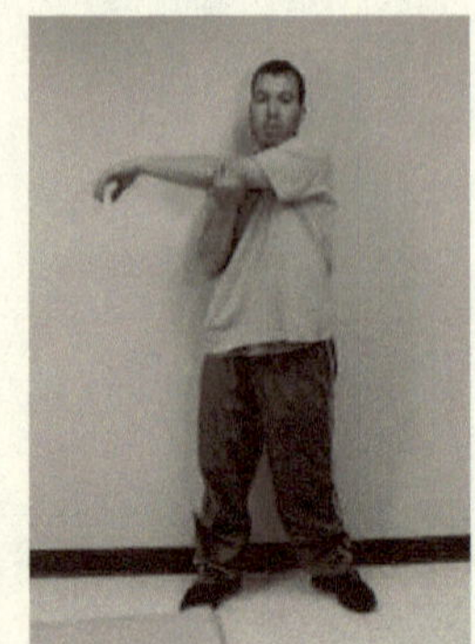

Stand straight. Spread your feet shoulder-distance apart. Grasp your right elbow with your left hand. Slowly pull your right arm to your left as far as possible. Hold this position for about five seconds. Repeat this process with left arm.

Biceps Stretch

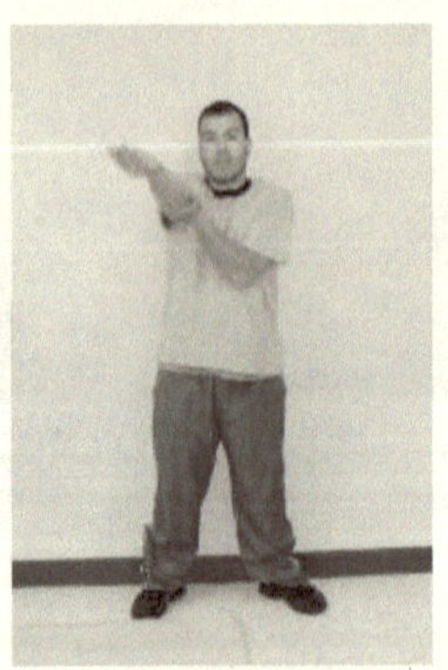
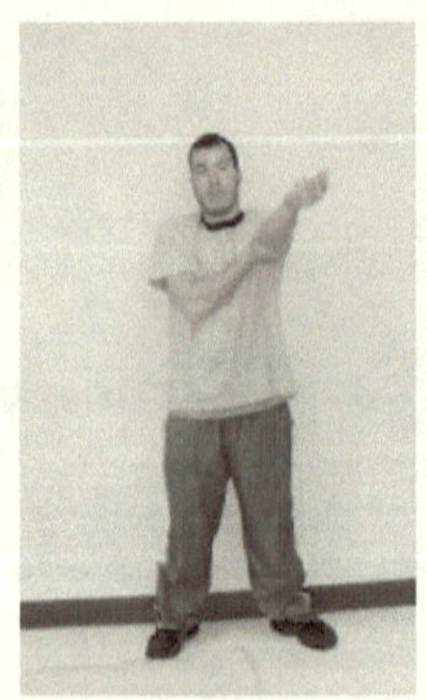

Stand straight. Spread your feet shoulder-distance apart. With palm facing up, extend right arm forward. Straighten your arm outward while placing your left hand underneath your elbow. Press your elbow down into your left hand and hold for about five seconds. Repeat this process with your right arm.

Exercise

Now that you have stretched your different muscle groups, you are ready to do some resistance exercise. You can start with the hardest and work your way to the easiest. Try the following exercises:

Cobra Span

Strengthens lower back and can help align spine.

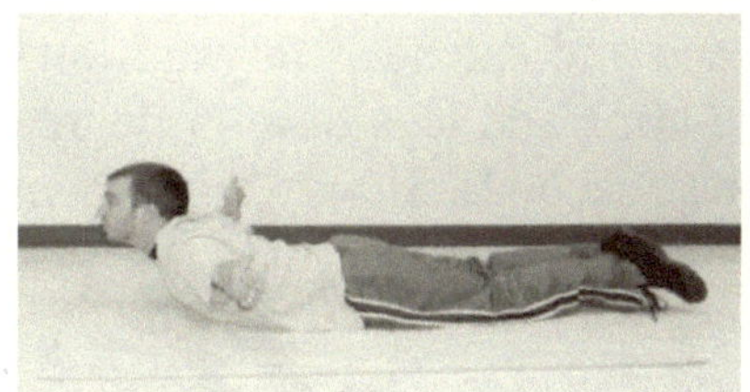

Lie flat on the floor face down. Extend both arms outward with your thumbs up and palms facing forward. Lift your head as far as you can while raising both arms and bringing shoulder blades together.

Hold for four counts, then relax. Do 15 repetitions.

Back Roll

Works the back muscles and can help your posture.

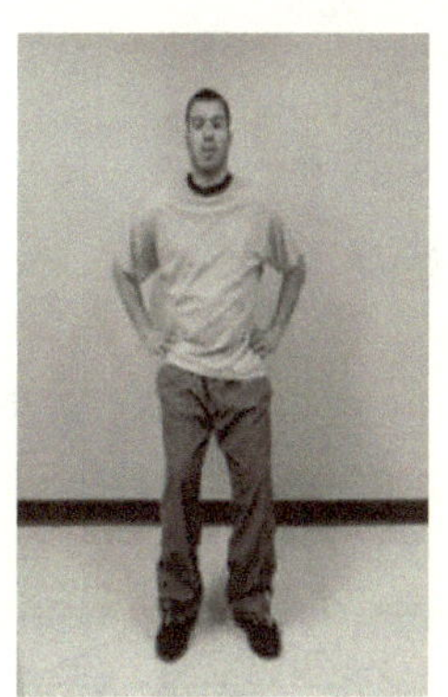

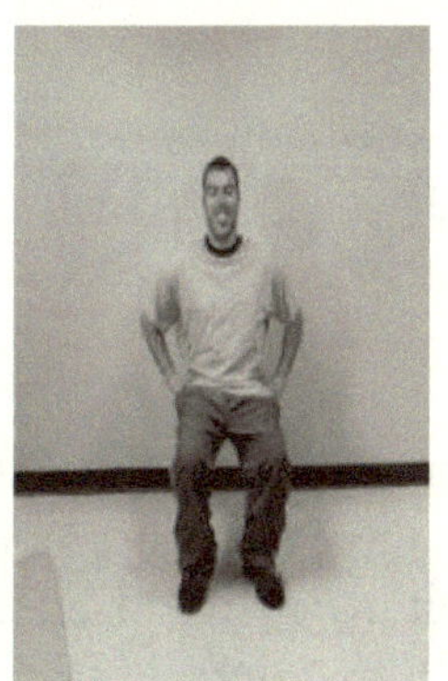

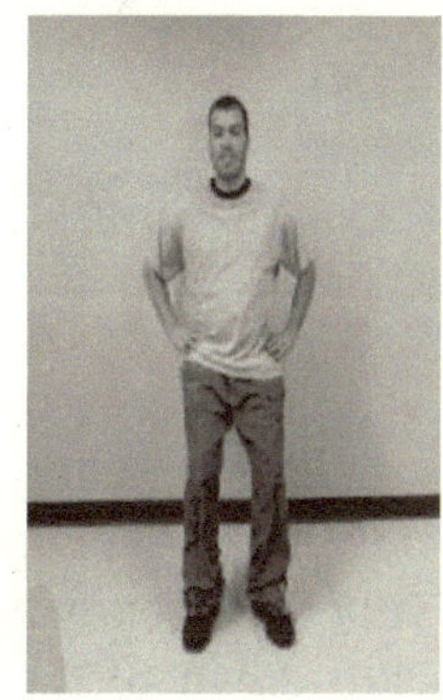

Place an exercise ball (not visible in this photo) on your back against the wall. Place your hands on your hips. Bend your knees as if you were going to sit and let the ball roll to your upper back. Count to four and stand while letting the ball roll to your upper back. Do 15 repetitions.

Arm and Leg Raise

Works the abdominal muscles.

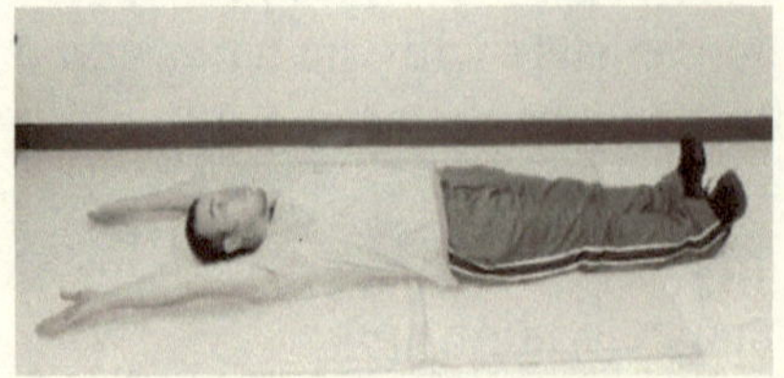
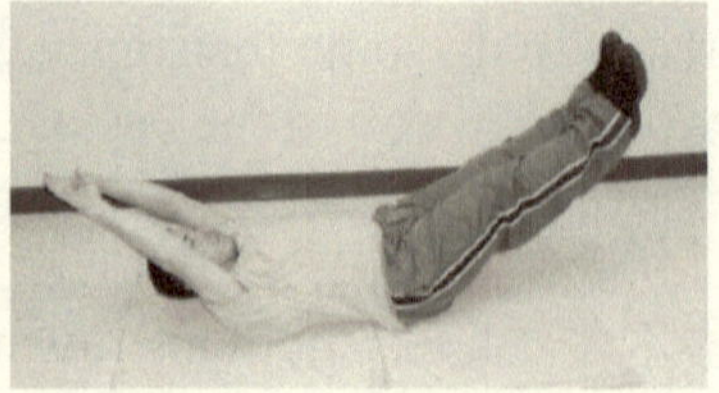

Lie flat on your back with legs closed and extended forward, and stretch both arms over your head. Raise arms and legs to a 45-degree angle at the same time. Keep them up for 10 seconds. Slowly bring them down. Do 15 repetitions.

Push-ups

Works the back, shoulder, triceps, chest, and abdominal muscles and promotes body strength.

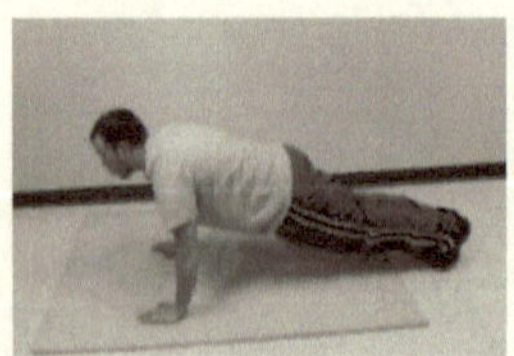
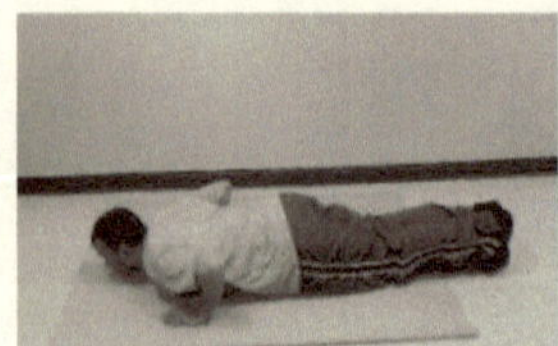
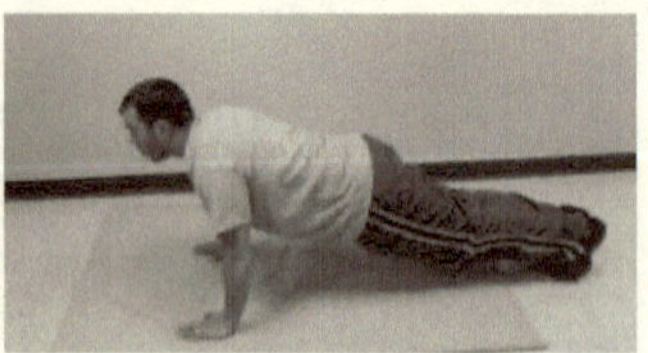

Drop to a horizontal or prone position. Stretch your arms in a vertical position with palms flat on the floor. Keep your body straight and support your lower body weight with your toes. Bending your elbows, bring your chin down to the floor. Push yourself back up by straightening your elbows. You can start with at least 10 and then increase the count as your body gets used to this exercise.

Sit-ups

Basic abdominal stretch that helps tone the abdominal muscles.

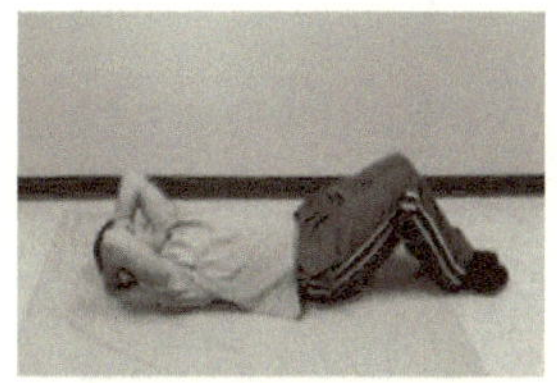
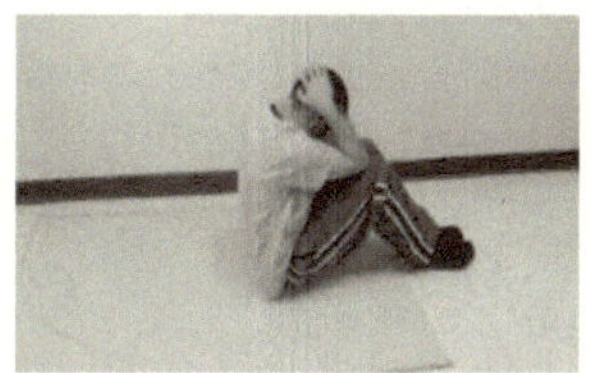
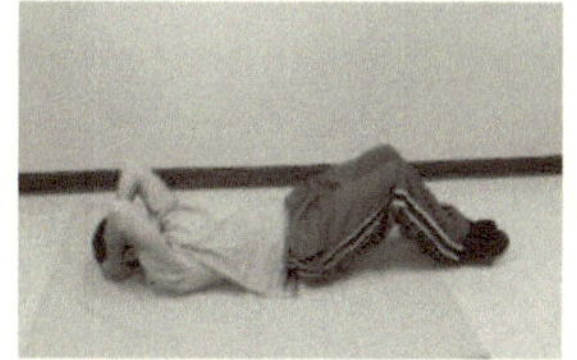

Lie flat on your back, put both hands behind your head, and lock your fingers behind your neck. Bring elbows as close together as possible. Bend your knees with your feet flat on the floor. Bring your head up until your elbows touch your knees. Slowly bring your head back down to the floor. Do as many as you can until you can feel your stomach tightening. Increase the number of sit-ups as you work out each day.

Crunches

If you cannot do full sit-ups you can start with crunches. This will work the same group of muscles as the sit-ups.

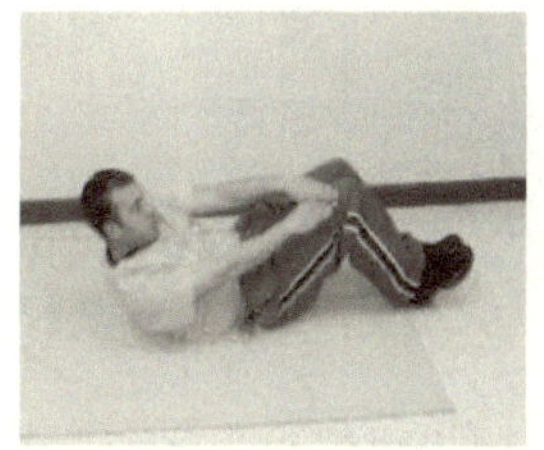
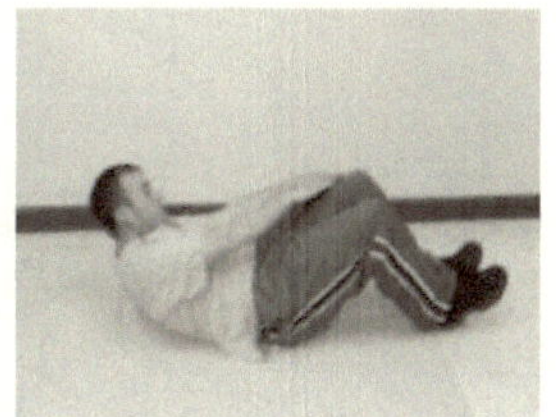
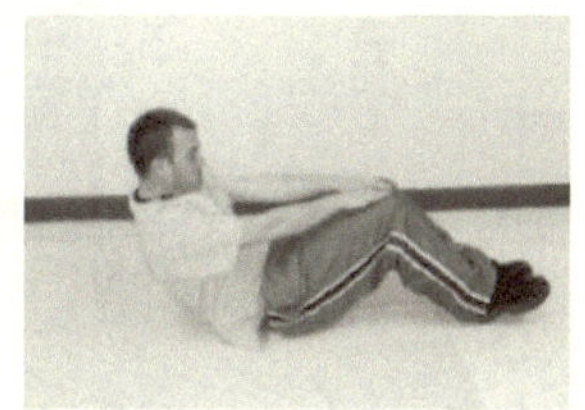

Lie flat on your back; bring your arms forward and hands together to form a triangle. Bend your knees and keep your feet flat on the floor. Raise your hands, and bring them to the right side of your legs for four counts. Go to your left leg for four counts and then to your knees for four counts. Do 15 repetitions.

Side Bends

Stretches and tones oblique (love handles).

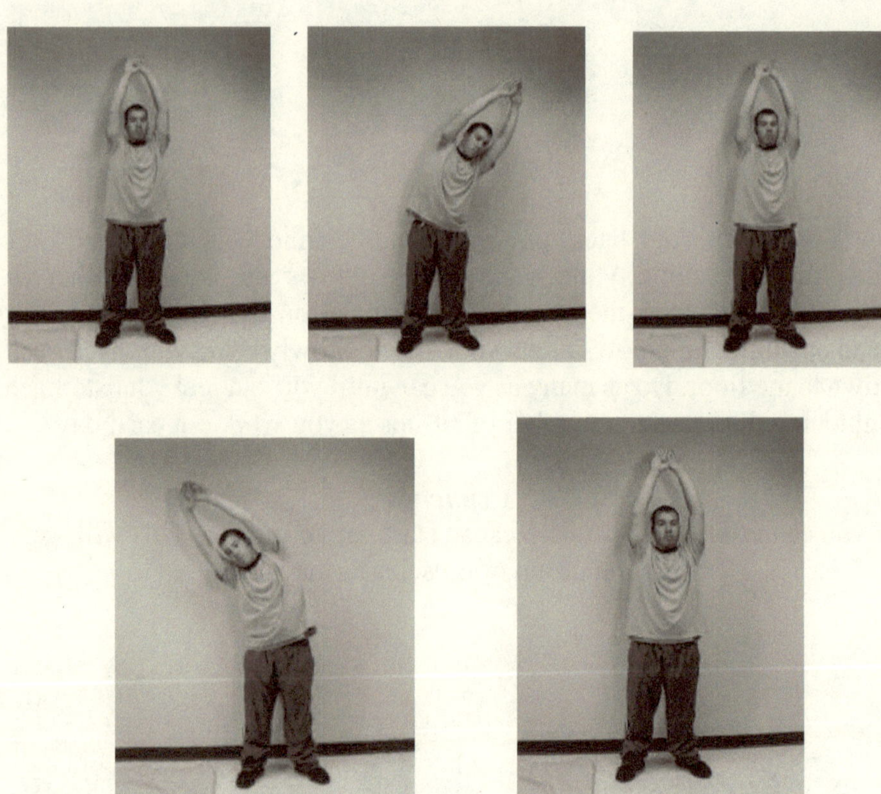

With your feet spread at shoulder distance, bring your arms up vertically. Put your hands together over your head to form a triangle. Bend toward the left side as far as possible for four counts. Straighten your body, and then bend to the right side as far as possible for four counts. Go back to the starting position. Do 15 repetitions.

Standing Squats

Works the quads and gives overall leg strength. Make sure that knees do not go past the toes. Keep stomach in and back as straight as possible.

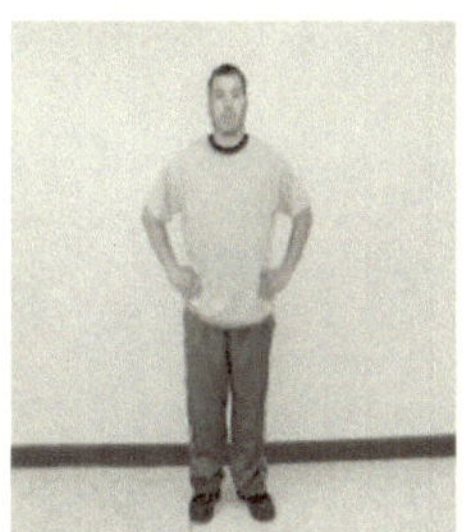
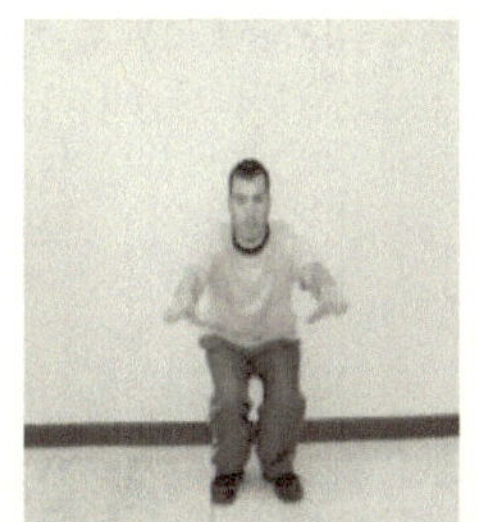
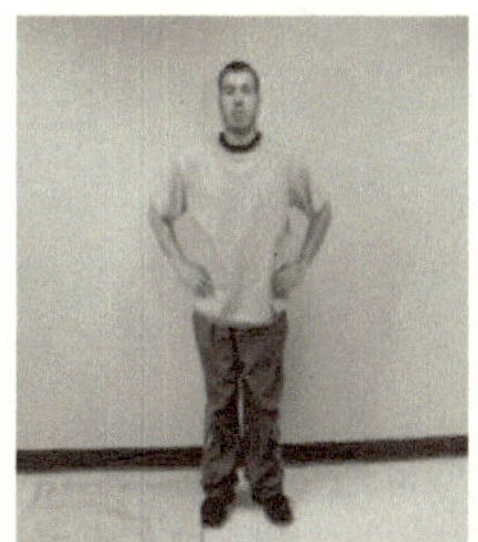

Stand straight with both hands on hips, and spread legs to a shoulder distance. Bend your legs, and go into a sitting position while stretching your arms forward and parallel to the floor. Straighten your legs, and go back to a standing position while putting your hands back on your hips. Do 15 repetitions.

Lateral Leg Raise

This exercise works and tones the abdominal muscles.

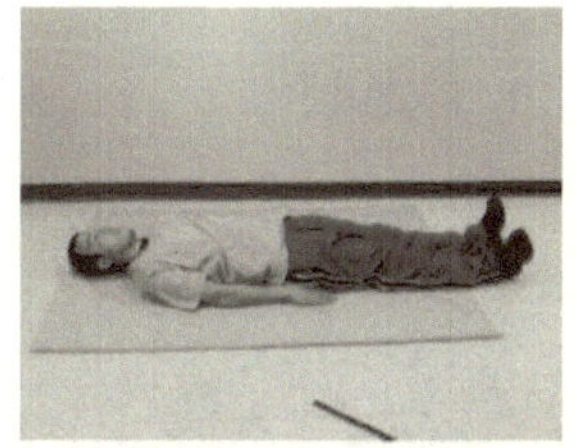
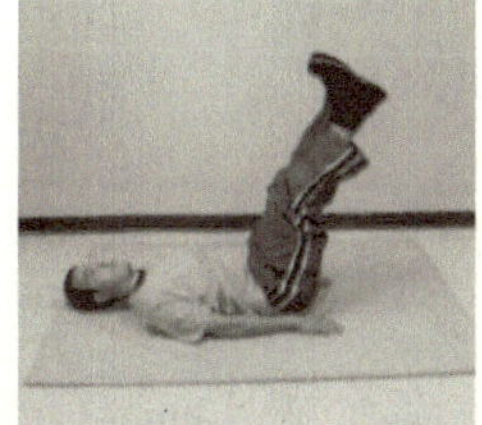
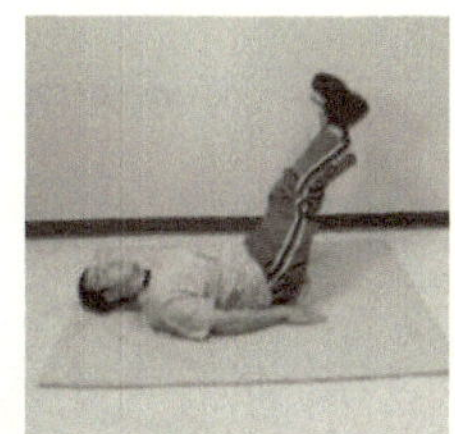
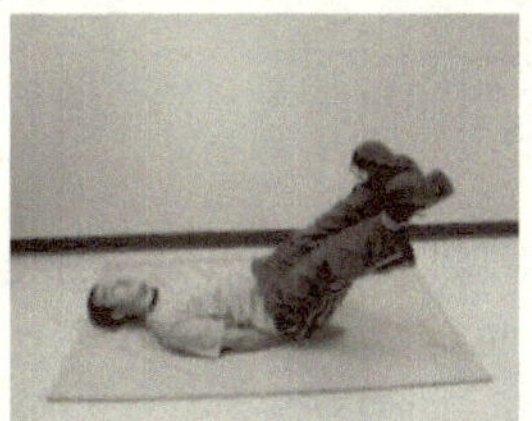
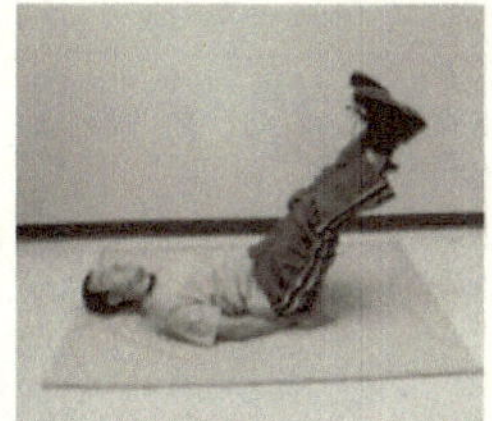

Lie flat on your back with arms flat on the floor; raise your legs to a 45 degree angle. Bring your legs together to the left for four counts.

Bring legs to starting positions, and then go to your right for four counts. Do 15 repetitions.

If you have a set of dumbbells you can do the following exercises.

Arm Curls

This exercise works and firms the biceps

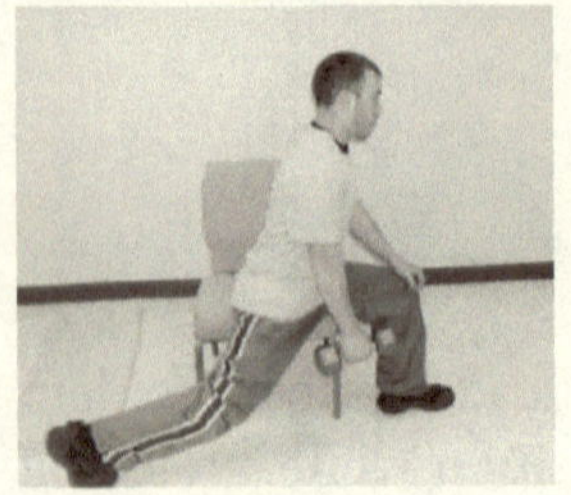
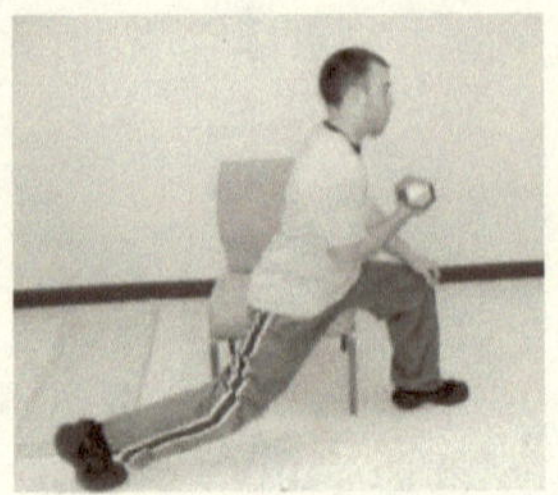
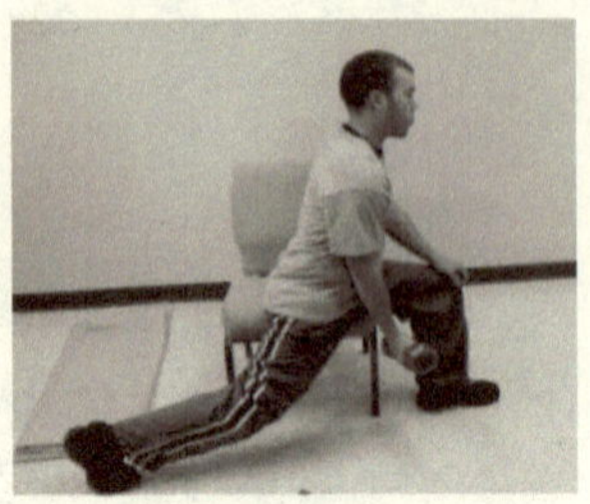

With your left leg bent and resting on a chair and your right leg supporting your weight, bring your right arm down to pick up the dumbbell. Bend your elbow gradually to lift the dumbbell as high as you can. Gradually lower your hand for four counts. Switch hands, and repeat exercise. Do 15 repetitions.

Parallel Arm Raise

Works the deltoids and small muscles of the shoulder.

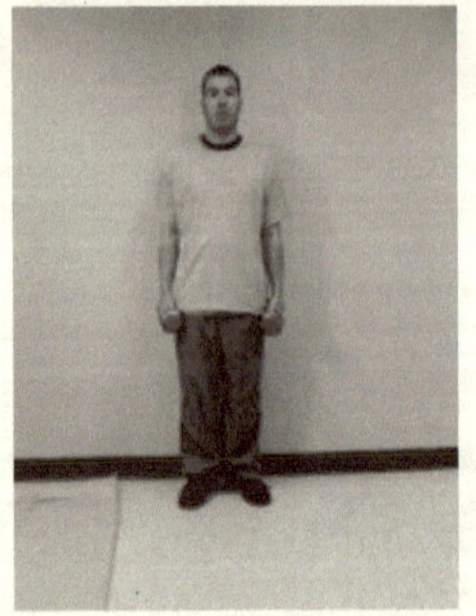
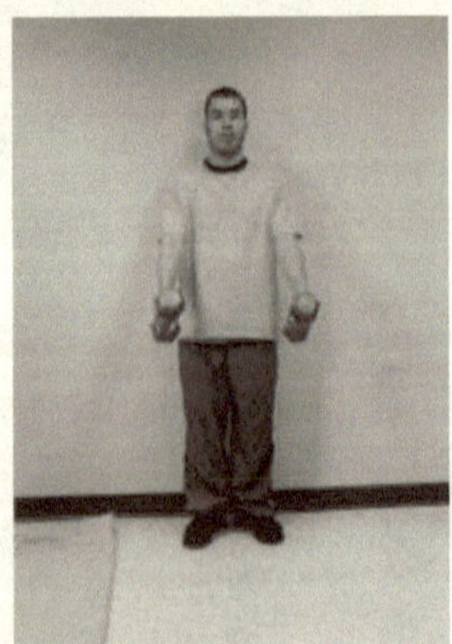
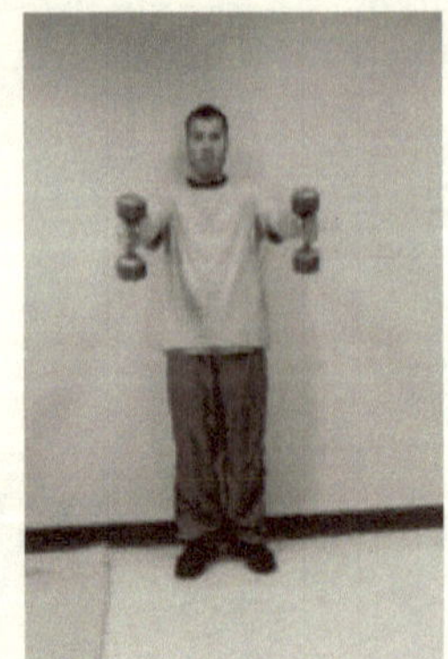

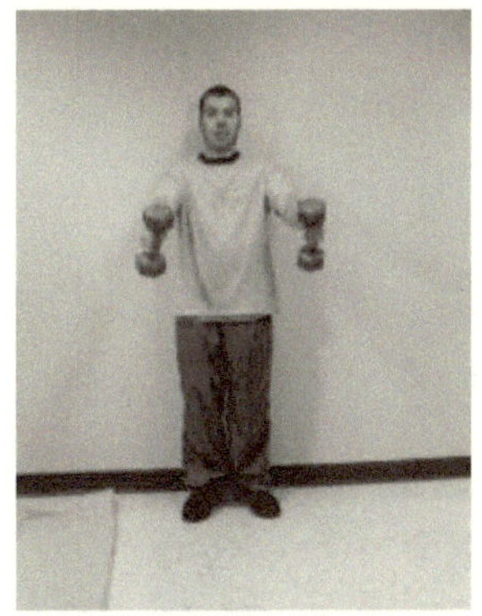
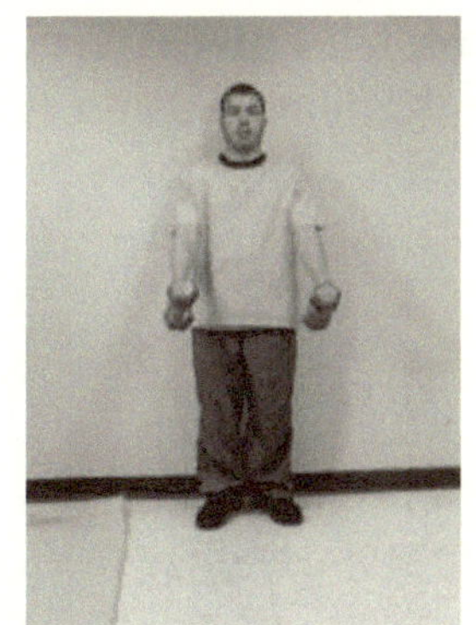
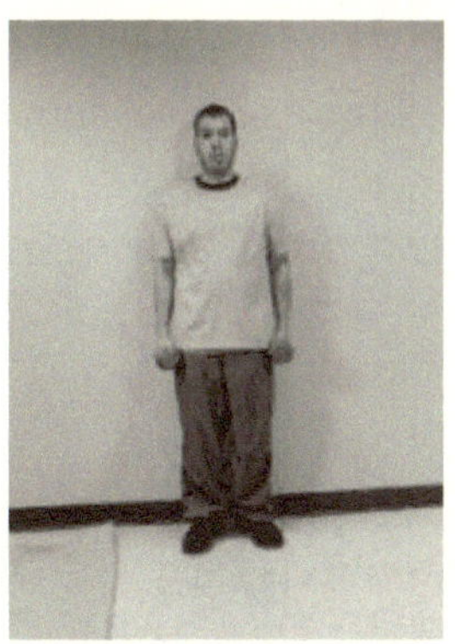

Stand straight, stomach in, chest out, shoulders back. Take a dumbbell in each hand. Put your hands by your side. Bring your arms up slowly in front of you for four counts until your arms are horizontal and parallel to the floor. Hold it for a few seconds, and then let your hands drop slowly for four counts until your hands are down to your sides. Do 15 repetitions.

Dumbbell Arm Raise

This exercise also works the deltoids and the outer portion of the pectorals (chest muscles).

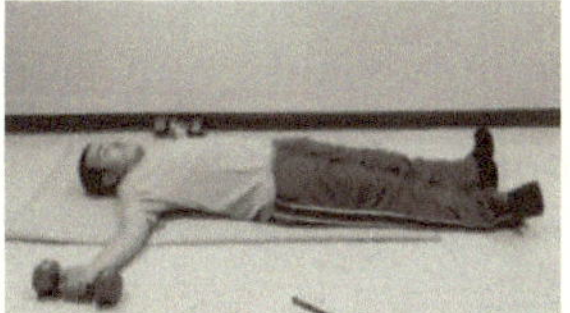
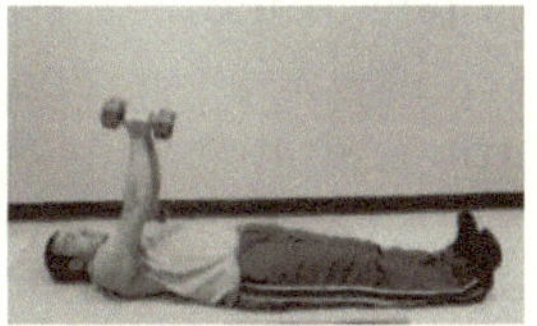
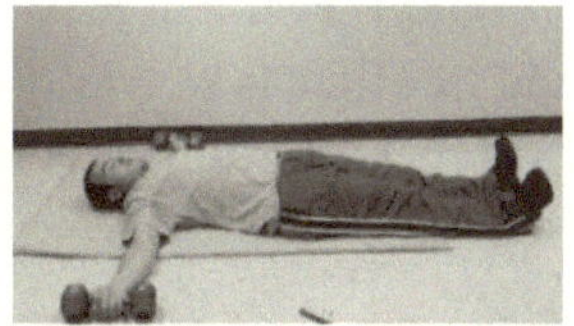

Begin by lying flat on your back on the floor or a bench. With a dumbbell in each hand, extend your arms outward. With your arms extended, bring dumbbells together to the point where they touch. Lower your arms, and repeat for four counts. Do 15 repetitions.

Dumbbell Lateral Arm Raise

This exercise, same as the dumbbell arm raise, emphasizes the back muscles.

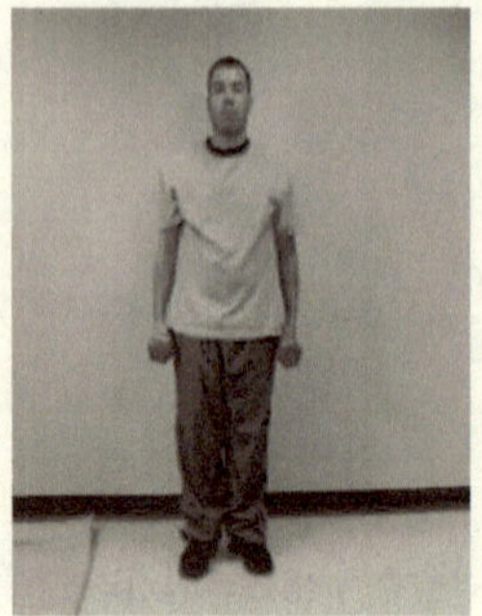

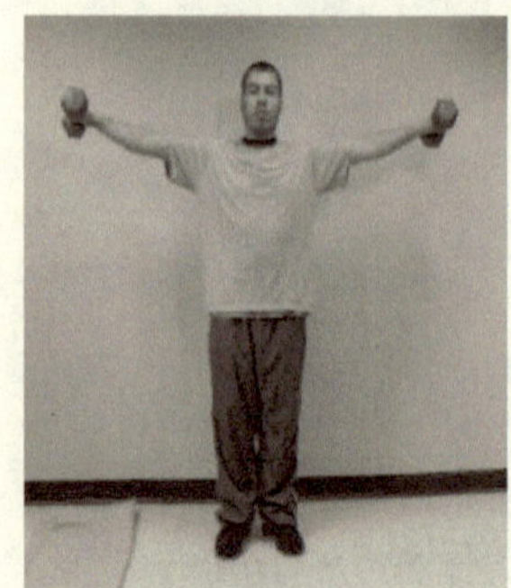

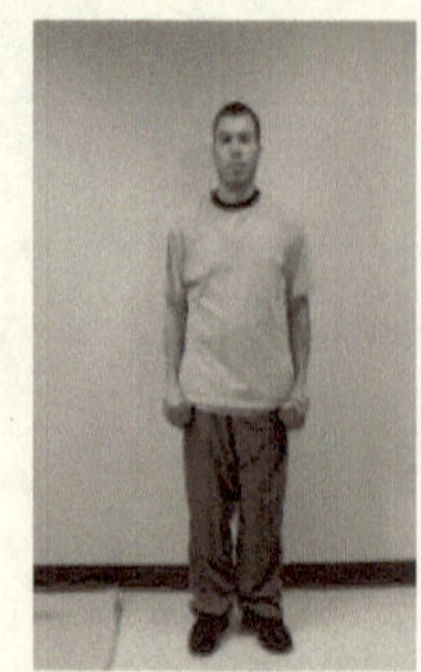

Stand straight, stomach in, chest out, shoulders back. Take a dumbbell in each hand. Put your hands to your side. With palms clutching your dumbbells facing down, extend your arms straight outward, bringing them up slowly until they are parallel to the floor. Hold that position for a few seconds and then lower your arms slowly. Do that for four counts. Do 15 repetitions.

These are just some of many exercises you can fit into your basic workout schedule. You can do them all in one day or combine some with walking. You can also do a few of these resistance exercises in one day and another few sets of exercises another day. The important thing is to exercise all your muscle groups so that your body can tone evenly.

Walking Exercise

Walking is one of the best fat-burning exercises you can do. Doctors recommend that you walk for at least 30 minutes a day, five times a week. Besides burning fat, walking will help your blood circulate. If you are hypertensive or diabetic, walking will help bring down your weight and control your blood pressure and diabetes. Walking plays an important role in the prevention of heart disease.

Some people find exercise boring and painful, which is why getting started is hard. However, once you start to do a little each day you will soon get into the habit. Some experts say that it takes 21 days for your body to adapt to anything. That is why getting started is very important. Remember, a little exercise is better than no exercise at all. Exercise need not be boring or painful. Perhaps you have a friend that you can invite to walk with you, or maybe you can make walking a time for prayer, reflection, or meditation. You might even want to buy an iPod so that you can listen to your favorite music while you walk. Seek the best way possible to make walking something you will enjoy. If you walk on your treadmill, you might try what I do. I usually turn on the television or read a book. That takes my mind away from the exercise and makes time go by faster.

The best way to start exercising is by walking. When you begin any exercise program start gradually. Start out by walking at least 15 minutes a day. As you adapt you can increase your time and distance. Instead of a half mile a day, you can step up to three quarters of a mile. Instead of 15 minutes, you can advance to 25 and so on. Before you realize it, you will be going the distance. Do not push yourself to the limits when you are just starting. As I have mentioned a few times in this section, you do not want to do too much too soon. If you are going to walk or jog, you will need to start at a slow to moderate pace. The idea is to work your way into exercising. After a few weeks, you can increase your speed. You could start by walking for 15 minutes and running for five. Later on you could walk for five and run for 10 minutes. You could combine your walking and jogging – however you feel comfortable. Always remember to check your pulse frequently during your workout. You need to accelerate your heart rate to a higher level for a good cardiovascular workout.

Don't forget to cool down before you quit your exercise for the day. Your cool-down period is also your recovery phase. It helps slow down your breathing and gradually brings down your heart rate. Once you have cooled down, it is important to stretch those muscles you have just worked. If you fail to do that you are likely to be in for a lot of pain for the next few days.

Weekly Exercise Schedule

I would suggest that you make a contract with yourself and commit yourself to an exercise program that fits your schedule. Your exercise schedule could look like this:

Monday	Tuesday	#	Wednesday	Thursday	#	Friday
Stretches	Stretches	15	Stretches	Stretches	15	Stretches
Walk 30-60 minutes	Push-ups	*	Walk 30-60 minutes	Crunches	15	Walk 30-60 minutes
	Sit-ups	*		Arm and Leg Raise	15	
	Arm Curls	15		Parallel Arm Raise	15	
	Cobra Span	15		D-bell Lateral Arm Raise	15	
	D-bell Arm Raise	15		Sit-ups	*	
	Back Roll	15		Push-ups	*	
	Side Bends	15		Knee Bends	15	
	Standing Squats	15		Lateral leg Raise	15	

\# Repetition * As many as you are able

Chart – By the author

You can add Saturday to your schedule combining resistance exercise and walking. You can make your own schedule by adding other exercises. However, be sure to cover all of the muscle groups during that week.

Getting started with exercise is not easy. It takes motivation and will power. One motivator would be seeing the results of your hard work and feeling better about yourself. However, you will not see any results if you do not begin. So stop procrastinating and making excuses, and get started.

This exercise program is not limited to clergy members; however, they are the ones responsible for educating their congregations, not just in spiritual matters but in matters of physical health as well. I recommend that pastors take initiative in caring for their own health, and then promote good health care in their local church. To do otherwise would be like preaching to the choir. The exercise program that I have discussed in this book can be part of a church program where pastors can facilitate and participate in it together with their church members. This way pastors can lead by example and grow healthy together with the people whom they are called to serve.

Live Healthy, Live Longer

God has created us to live long, healthy, and productive lives. God's good intention is for us to be healthy in every aspect of our lives. God has made us accountable for the proper care of our body, mind, and spirit. We are to be good stewards of all that God has given us, including our health. A healthy body can increase our chances of living longer and having the energy to carry out the mission God has called us to do.

As pastors, we are responsible not just for the spiritual well-being of our congregations, but for their physical and emotional well-being as well. To care for our congregations, however, we must first care for our own spiritual, physical, and emotional health. We need to invest our time and energy to be in optimum condition so that we can effectively lead and care for our congregations, not as wounded healers, but as healthy caregivers.

Health and wholeness are necessary for clergy members if they are to function properly and effectively in ministry. That is why it is important for pastors to care for themselves while caring for their congregations. That means taking care of our health in three dimensions; spirit, mind, and body.

NOTES

1. *The Greek New Testament. Third corrected edition* 1983. United Bible Societies.
2. Steinke, Peter L. *How Your Church Family Works: Understanding Congregations as Emotional Systems*. Herndon, VA: The Alban Institute, 1993. p. 4.
3. Wagner, James K. *An Adventure in Healing and Wholeness: The Healing Ministry of Christ in the Church Today*. Nashville, TN : Upper Room Books, 1993. p. 11. Quote from David Hilton's speech "Ethics, Worldview, and Health," an address to the American Public Health Association, 117th Annual Meeting (1989).
4. Slaughter, Michael. *Momentum for Life: Sustaining Personal Health, Integrity, and Strategic focus as a Leader*. Nashville, TN: Abingdon Press, 2005. p. 46.
5. Ibid., p. 45.
6. UNCF (1972-Present). 1972. http:/stagingadcouncil.org./default.aspx.
7. Soukanov, Anne H. et al. *Encarta World English Dictionary*. New York: St. Martin's Press, 1999.
8. Ibid.
9. Savant, Marilyn vos and Fleischer, Lenore. *Brain Building: Exercising Yourself Smarter*. New York: Bantam Books, 1990. p. vii.
10. Soukanov, op. cit.
11. Ibid.
12. Bradshaw, John. *Healing the Shame That Binds You*. Dearfield Beach FL : Health Communications Inc, 1988. p. 17.
13. Ibid. p. vii.
14. Ibid.
15. Smedes, Lewis. *Shame and Grace: Healing the Shame We Don't Deserve*. San Francisco : Zondervon Publishing House, 1993. p. 34.
16. Bradshaw, op.cit., p. 10.
17. Ibid. p. 17.
18. Bradshaw, op. cit., p. 61.
19. Erikson, Erik H. *Identity and the Life Cycle*. New York : W.W. Norton & Co., 1959. p. 52.

20. Alexander, Neil M, [ed.]. *The United Methodist Book of Discipline*. Nashville, TN : United Methodist Publishing House, 2008. p. 235.
21. Butler, Gillian and Hope, Tony. *Managing Your Mind: The Mental Fitness Guide*. New York : Oxford University Press, 2007. p. 89.
22. Ibid. p. 90.
23. Ibid. p. 97.
24. Seamands, David A. *Healing for Damaged Emotions*. Wheaton, Il: Victor Books, a Division of Scripture Press Publications, Inc., 1988. p. 49.
25. Butler and Hope, op. cit. p. 95.
26. Ibid. p. 254.
27. Ibid.
28. Rubin, Jordan and Remedios, David M. *The Great Physicians Rx for Health and Wellness: Seven Keys to Unlock Your Health Potential.* Nashville, TN: Thomas Nelson Books, 2005. p. 205.
29. Ibid., p. x.
30. Ibid. p. ix.
31. Slaughter, Michael. op. cit. p. 146.
32. Rubin, Jordan S. op. cit. p. 148
33. Ibid.
34. Ford-Martin, Paula and Blumer, Ian. *The Everything Diabetes Book.* Avon, MA : Adams Media Corp, 2004. p. 11.
35. Ibid. p. 21.
36. Alterman, Seymour L., and Kullman Donald A. *Diabetes: Prevention, Control, and Cure*. Frederick Fell, 2000. p. 153.
37. Chasnoff, Ira J., Ellis, Jeffrey W., Fainman, Zachary. *Family Medical Guide*. Lincolnwood, Il: Publications International Ltd, 1983. p. 206.
38. Ford-Martin and Blumer. op. cit. p. 169.
39. Alvarez, Manny, MD. Obesity in Children. Fox News Channel, New York : Hemmer, Bill, May 2006.
40. Rubin, Jordan. op. cit. p. xxiii.
41. Alterman and Kullman, op. cit. p. 148.
42. Ibid.
43. Ibid.
44. Ibid. p. 150.
45. Ibid.

46. Ibid. p. 155.
47. Ibid. p. 151.
48. Ibid. p. 152.
49. Ibid.
50. Saudek, Christopher D., Rubin, Richard R., and Shump, Cynthia. *The Johns Hopkins Guide to Diabetes: For Today and Tomorrow*. Baltimore: The Johns Hopkins University Press, 1997. p. 116.
51. Ibid.
52. Alterman, Seymour L., and Kullman, Donald, A. *Diabetes: Prevention, Control, and Cure*. Frederick Fell Publishers Inc. 2000. p. 154
53. Saudek, Rubin, and Shump. op. cit. p. 126.
54. Alterman, and Kullman, op. cit. p. 238.
55. Ibid.
56. Caprio, Sonia MD. Diabetes Spectrum. [Online] October 2003. [Cited: October 6, 2012.] http://spectrum.diabetesjournal.or/content/16/4/230.fill.
57. Saudek, Rubin, and Shump. op. cit. p. 29.
58. Ibid. p. 113.
59. Ibid. p. 139.
60. Ibid. p. 140.

BIBLIOGRAPHY

Alexander, Neil M, [ed.]. (2008). *The United Methodist Book of Discipline*. Nashville, TN : United Methodist Publishing House.

Alterman, Seymour L., and Kullman, Donald A. *Diabetes: Prevention, Control, and Cure.* New York: Frederick Fell Publishers, Inc.

Alvarez, Manny, MD. Obesity in Children. Fox News Channel, New York : Hemmer, Bill, May 2006.

Bradshaw, John (1988). *Healing the Shame That Binds You.* Dearfield Beach, FL: Health Communications Inc.

Butler, Gillian, and Hope, Tony (2007) 2nd Edition. *Managing Your Mind: The Mental Fitness Guide*. New York: Oxford University Press.

Caprio, Sonia MD. Diabetes Spectrum. [Online] October 2003. Cited: October 6, 2012. http://spectrum.diabetesjournal.or/content/16/4/230.fill.

Chasnoff, Ira J., Ellis, Jeffrey W., and Fainman, Zachary S. (1983). *Family Medical Guide*. Lincolnwood, IL: Publications International Ltd.

Erikson, Erik H. (1959). *Identity and the Life Cycle*. New York: W.W. Norton & Co.

Ford-Martin, Paula, and Blumer, Ian (2004). *The Everything Diabetes Book.* Avon, MA: Adams Media Corp.

Kurt Aland, et al., [ed.]. (1983). *The Greek New Testament*. Third (Corrected). Federal Republic of Germany: The United Bible Society.

Merriam-Webster's Collegiate© Dictionary, 11th Edition ©2013 by Merriam-Webster, Inc. (www.Merriam-Webster.com)

Olson, Harriett Jane (Ed.) (2004). *The Book of Discipline of The United Methodist Church.* Nashville, TN: The United Methodist Publishing House.

Rubin, Jordan S.and Remedios, David M. (2005). *The Great Physicians Rx for Health and Wellness: Seven Keys to Unlock Your Health Potential.* Nashville, TN: Thomas Nelson Books.

Saudek, Christopher D., Rubin, Richard R., and Shump, Cynthia (1997). *The Johns Hopkins Guide to Diabetes: For Today and Tomorrow*. Baltimore: The Johns Hopkins University Press.

Savant, Marilyn vos, and Fleischer, Leonore (1990). *Brain Building: Exercising Yourself Smarter*. New York: Bantam Books.

Seamands, David A. (1988). *Healing for Damaged Emotions*. Wheaton, IL: Victor Books, a Division of Scripture Press Publications Inc.

Slaughter, Michael (2005). *Momentum for Life: Sustaining Personal Health, Integrity, and Strategic Focus as a Leader*. Nashville, TN: Abingdon Press.

Smedes, Lewis B. (1993). *Shame and Grace: Healing the Shame We Don't Deserve*. San Francisco: Zondervon Publishing House.

Soukanov, Anne H. et al. (1999). *Encarta World English Dictionary*. New York : St. Martin's Press.

Steinke, Peter L. (1993). *How Your Church Family Works: Understanding Congregations as Emotional Systems*. Herndon, VA: The Alban Institute.

UNCF 1972-Present.(Online) 1972. www.aes.com

Wagner, James K. (1993). *An Adventure in Healing and Wholeness: The Healing Ministry of Christ in the Church Today*. Nashville, TN: Upper Room.

www.ingramcontent.com/pod-product-compliance
Lightning Source LLC
LaVergne TN
LVHW051011080826
845145LV00009B/2573

* 9 7 8 0 9 3 4 9 5 5 9 4 2 *